GW00320010

John Hunter is a Consultant Physician at Addenbrooke's Hospital, Cambridge and a recognized authority on the subject of food allergy and intolerance. He developed an interest in food in relation to diseases of the gut in response to the need of the many sufferers of irritable bowel syndrome attending his out-patients' clinic. He has contributed over 40 research papers to major medical journals including the *Lancet, Update* and the *British Medical Journal.*

Virginia Alun Jones has been research fellow to Dr Hunter at Addenbrooke's since 1982. As well as contributing to this book, she has presented the results of the team's work at scientific meetings in this country and Europe. She too has written numerous articles for among others the *British Medical Journal,* the *Lancet,* and the *Journal of the Royal College of General Practitioners.*

Elizabeth Workman gained her State Registration as a dietitian after following the dietetics course at Leeds Polytechnic, already being a holder of a biological sciences degree from Leicester University. She has gained great expertise in helping people with food-related diseases over the last 4 years and enjoys the challenge of devising appetizing and nutritious recipes from unusual ingredients, not least because her husband is a vegetarian and she caters for a growing family.

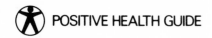
POSITIVE HEALTH GUIDE

THE
ALLERGY
DIET

How to overcome your food intolerance

Elizabeth Workman, SRD
Dr John Hunter
Dr Virginia Alun Jones

MARTIN DUNITZ

© Dr John Hunter, Dr Virginia Alun Jones and Mrs Elizabeth Workman SRD, 1984

First published in the United Kingdom in 1984
by Martin Dunitz Ltd, 154 Camden High Street, London NW1 0NE

British Library Cataloguing in Publication Date

Jones, Virginia Alun
   The allergy diet.—(Positive health guide)
   1. Food allergy
   I. Title II. Hunter, John, 19--
   III. Workman, Elizabeth IV. Series
   616.97'5 RC596
ISBN 0-906348-69-2
ISBN 0-906348-70-6 (pbk)

Phototypeset in Garamond by Book Ens, Saffron Walden, Essex

Printed by Toppan Printing Company (S) Pte Ltd, Singapore

Reprinted 1984

Front cover photograph shows: Strawberry ice (top right, see page 106), Feta salad (top left, see page 55), Apple and walnut teabread and Bread rolls bottom left, see pages 92 and 91), Roast chicken (bottom right, see page 74)

Back cover photograph shows: The devil's own drumsticks (top, see page 65), Apple and bean salad (bottom, see page 52)

CONTENTS

INTRODUCTION

Food allergy is a term that the medical profession is wary of, and rightly so. A great deal of press coverage has led to the popular idea that any number of foods from avocado pear to zucchini can cause a whole range of 'allergic' reactions including rashes, runny noses, headaches. This has meant that people have been diagnosing all sorts of food allergies for themselves and may be in danger of nutritional deficiencies by excluding too many foods from their diets.

In this book we show how a number of conditions are known to be caused by intolerance to particular foods. We and other researchers have proved by medical trials that this food intolerance can be treated by putting people on to a diet excluding the ingredients that cause their symptoms. The diets need careful balancing to ensure that they are properly nutritious and healthy, and from our menu plans and recipes you will see that they can also be made appetizing and attractive.

Unfortunately the foods that cause the conditions vary from person to person and discovering the true culprits can be time consuming and difficult. Few doctors at present have experience in this new field, so we have written this book to help people with various symptoms – and their doctors – establish whether or not they do have a food intolerance and, if so, how to deal with it.

What is allergy?

Most of the books written about food and disease call the condition 'food allergy'. Originally the word allergy meant an unpleasant reaction to any foreign substance in the body, but over the years it has changed, and now doctors use it to describe a reaction caused by a breakdown of the immune system.

The real job of the immune system is to recognize and destroy infecting agents such as bacteria and viruses that have got into the body. Substances in the blood called antibodies are produced and these make the cells defending the body attack the germs. In allergic reactions an abnormal type of antibody is produced that reacts to certain foreign substances called allergens, such as spores, pollens and foods. The combination of these antibodies with the allergen produces the allergic symptoms.

In most allergies doctors can detect the allergic reaction going on in the blood, but in the case of food allergy this type of reaction is hardly ever found. This is why doctors have doubted the existence of such a condition as food allergy. Yet some foods have been proved to cause disease.

How do foods produce diseases?

We are still unsure of the way that these foods cause symptoms.

We do know that some contain chemicals that upset some people but not others. Milk, for example, contains a sugar called lactose which is digested by a natural chemical called an enzyme, found in the wall of the intestine. All children have this enzyme but it disappears in all but the white races in early adult life. This means that many people develop diarrhoea if they drink milk, because they are unable to break down the lactose.

We have now found that one of the reasons why some people react to chemicals is probably linked to the way the various enzymes in their bodies behave. A clue in the discovery was the action of one of the enzymes called mono-amine oxidase. Certain drugs reduce its activity, and people who are taking them have to avoid eating foods such as cheese, red wine, yeast or yeast extract, otherwise they get high blood pressure and severe headaches.

Unfortunately, it is not as simple as that – food intolerance is not always the result of the enzymes' behaviour. There are other chemicals that work in different ways, including caffeine, histamine and tyramine. Caffeine is found in tea, coffee, cocoa, cola drinks and chocolate; histamine in cheese, beer, sausages and canned foods; and tyramine in brewer's yeast, red wine and cheese. Too much strong coffee produces many familiar symptoms – restlessness, palpitations, and heartburn. Histamine and tyramine may be a cause of migraine. It is thought that when they are absorbed into the body they may change the diameter of small blood vessels, and so bring on an attack in people who get migraine.

In our research in Cambridge we have found that many people who cannot eat wheat release large amounts of histamine from the lining of their intestine when wheat comes in contact with it – perhaps they have special cells there which produce this reaction.

People often develop the irritable bowel syndrome (see opposite) after a bout of gastroenteritis or repeated courses of antibiotics. We have now found that many with the condition have changes in the bacteria living in their intestines. It seems possible that these bacteria are responsible: they may break down food remnants to produce chemicals which cause the irritable bowel syndrome.

As there are so many different causes of reactions to food, and as most of them are nothing to do with allergy, you will see why we prefer to speak of 'food intolerance' rather than 'food allergy'.

Which conditions are caused by food intolerance?

As we explained, from the present state of knowledge about how foods cause disease, it can't be said that food intolerance is the cause in every case – there certainly are other known causes for all these conditions – but we and other researchers have shown by the success of our dietary treatment that food intolerance is the most common. If your child or you are diagnosed as having one of the diseases, a special diet is likely to be the remedy. But you must discuss this with your doctor, and if necessary a specialist, before you start excluding foods from your daily intake.

The conditions listed are the ones we have found are often caused by intolerance to one or other of the foods listed on page 19, and so are treated by a diet:

Irritable bowel syndrome
Migraine
Asthma
Rhinitis
Coeliac disease
Eczema
Urticaria
Cow's milk sensitive enteropathy

Recently we have also had a lot of success in Cambridge treating Crohn's disease (an inflammation of the intestine) by diet, but as this is still in the experimental stages and as the disease can be severe, any change in diet should be made only under close medical supervision at a hospital specializing in the condition.

Irritable bowel syndrome

Irritable bowel syndrome is a very common condition which affects twice as many women as men; nearly one person in three in the UK suffers from it to a greater or lesser extent at one time or another. It is also often known as spastic colon. The symptoms are bad abdominal pain and distension, together with diarrhoea or a very variable bowel habit. As we said earlier, people often develop symptoms after gastroenteritis or long courses of antibiotics. Yet the various x-rays and blood tests are always normal, and this has led many doctors to believe that the condition has psychological origins. People who have had abdominal pain for many years without relief tend to find life very stressful, but seeing a psychiatrist does not usually stop the symptoms, and our experience in Cambridge is that at least two-thirds of our patients suffering from irritable bowel syndrome have food intolerances. Of 182 patients treated by diet, we were able to relieve symptoms completely in 122. We wrote to eighty patients two years later to ask them how they were getting on. Seventy-one replied; fifty-nine were feeling well on their diet, and six were still well and had gone back to normal eating. So we have found treatment by diet to be far the best way of calming the irritable bowel.

Although not all cases are caused by food intolerance – menstrual changes can bring on the symptoms, and, less often, lack of fibre in the diet or short-term stress – we believe that anyone with irritable bowel syndrome should at least try an exclusion diet.

Migraine

Migraine is a very common problem, particularly in women – one woman in five between twenty and forty-five suffers from it. It has not yet been discovered why it should be so much more common in women. But migraine headaches do often run in families and usually affect only one side of the head at a time. Nausea and vomiting are associated symptoms. Attacks may last for as long as thirty-six or forty-eight hours, although many are much shorter. They seem to be brought on by a number of conditions, including tiredness, stress, excitement, fasting and bright lights as well as food.

Professor Soothill at Great Ormond Street, the famous children's hospital in London, takes a particular interest in treating migraine by diet. He found that of eighty-eight children who had at least one migraine a week, eighty-two were free from headaches after they had followed an exclusion diet, even when it had been thought that there were other causes. It was discovered that most of these children had a problem with four or fewer foods. Obviously it is fairly easy for children to avoid a small number of foods, and well worth while.

Asthma and rhinitis

Wheezing and difficulty in breathing are the main symptoms of asthma, and at night may be accompanied by coughing. There are a number of causes. It was found in one trial that some foods provoked asthma attacks in nearly 30 per cent of sufferers. Some people had only to smell the food to start an attack, although most of them actually had to eat it. Wheezing usually started an hour or two later. But food is only one cause of asthma, and as attacks can be serious, asthmatics in particular must discuss trying diet as treatment carefully with their doctors first.

Rhinitis is the medical name for a persistently runny or stuffy nose, and it can be, like asthma, related to food. Although the symptoms are so similar to a common cold, there is no confusion between the two since rhinitis doesn't come and go like a cold; it is a permanent condition. If your doctor has confirmed you have rhinitis it is certainly worth discussing trying a diet as treatment.

Coeliac disease

Coeliac disease affects about one in two to three thousand people in the UK, probably one in five thousand in the USA. It is a condition in which gluten, a protein found in wheat, rye and barley, damages the lining of the small intestine so that food is not properly absorbed. This leads to a number of difficulties including diarrhoea, bone disease and failure to grow, or loss of weight. Anaemia may also result from these problems. As the symptoms can be caused by several other conditions it is not safe to start a gluten-free diet as treatment without being diagnosed first by a specialist.

The discovery that coeliac disease was caused by gluten was

purely accidental. Most of the wheat grown in Holland during the Second World War was directed to the German army at the Front, so the civilian population had to make do with potatoes. At this time children with coeliac disease made dramatic improvements, and the Dutch specialist Dr W.K. Dicke made the connection, that excluding gluten from the diet had made the children better.

People with coeliac disease recover completely once they avoid foods containing gluten but they should still be seen regularly by their specialist to make sure they are well and not lapsing on the diet, even by mistake.

Commercial gluten-free products are available, but these are useful only to people with coeliac disease. Many of the recipes in this book are suitable for coeliacs and further help may be obtained from the national coeliac societies in the UK, North America and Australia.

Eczema

Eczema is an itching red rash, often on the insides of elbows and knees, which may scale and crust. It is common in both children and adults. The rash comes and goes. It is often treated by steroid creams and anti-histamine pills. Yet there is sound evidence that it can be caused by food intolerance, especially to eggs and milk. Fourteen out of twenty children tested at Great Ormond Street Hospital in London improved when cow's milk and eggs were taken out of their diet.

In another study at the University of Texas in the USA, thirty-two out of thirty-seven children with eczema improved after cow's milk was withdrawn from their diet and became worse when they were allowed to drink it again. The orange dye tartrazine which is found in yellow-coloured food (see page 16), is also often a cause of eczema. Food reactions produce changes in the blood, which suggests people with eczema have a genuine allergy.

Urticaria

This is a very common condition, especially in children. Large red itchy blotches appear anywhere on the skin. Other symptoms are swelling of the lips and mouth. Many factors can bring on urticaria including heat, light, pressure and vibration, but in 44 per cent of children who were tested, foods, artificial dyes, preservatives and additives were the reason. More recent studies have shown that salicylates (a chemical found in aspirin and in some foods), yeasts and cow's milk are also causes.

Cow's milk sensitive enteropathy

This mainly affects babies who are bottle-fed before the age of four months. The symptoms are the severe stomach pain known as colic, diarrhoea, eczema, vomiting and a runny nose. Babies usually grow out of these once they are on a solid diet, about the age of two.

Mothers who think their children are reacting to cow's milk should talk to their family doctors. Two or three simple tests (biopsies) on the small intestine while the baby is taking cow's milk and after it has been left off show whether or not that is the trouble. Although a cow's milk-free diet may be suggested for your baby by your doctor or paediatrician, never start a child on any abnormal diet without close medical supervision.

In the next part we explain how to find a diet that will relieve you of the symptoms caused by these conditions – as long of course as food intolerance is the reason in your case. Excluding foods may be hard to start with, but the test period is relatively short, and you'll probably find there are very few foods you have to cut out for long.

The diets

If you suffer from any of the symptoms we have described you may want to try a special diet. Discuss your symptoms beforehand with your doctor to make sure that he or she thinks this approach is sensible. You must be sure the doctor agrees that you have one of the conditions that can be treated by diet: it may be that you have another problem with similar symptoms but which needs different treatment. You should also discuss with your doctor whether or not you should continue with any pills or medicines that you may have been taking. In general it is better to take as few pills as possible whilst trying these diets, as many contain starches as fillers, and they may be part of the problem.

Vegetarians should think very carefully before deciding to follow a diet which may restrict the foods available to them. Unfortunately many of the foods which most commonly produce symptoms are those that are staple items for vegetarians, such as bread, milk, cheese and eggs.

The basic principle when trying an exclusion diet is to stop eating foods that are likely to upset you and to see if your symptoms get better. Any food can produce symptoms, although some do it much more frequently than others (see the table on page 19). Taking the treatment to extremes, you would begin by eating nothing at all. This is not, of course, a practical possibility at home. In severe cases of Crohn's disease we do stop people eating completely by feeding them with a drip until their symptoms have settled. But people with conditions such as migraine and irritable bowel syndrome are rarely ill enough to justify the great expense of this treatment.

Some doctors in the USA have advised people to live on water alone during this test period and others have suggested a diet limited to lamb and pears. We have tried these methods and now we hardly ever use them because they are both very unpleasant for the person concerned (physically and mentally) and nutritionally inadequate. Progress is slow because of the large number of foods that must be reintroduced later and if people have difficult food reactions it takes several weeks to arrange an adequate diet. Unless your doctor specifically recommends them, extreme exclusion diets are best avoided. Never try living on water alone unless in hospital under close supervision.

We prefer to keep our patients on wider diets, excluding only those foods which experience has shown are most likely to cause trouble. This may, of course, produce problems if people have unusual food intolerances but it seems to work much better for most people and we have had more overall success this way.

Which diet for which condition?

Once you have discovered what your intolerances are you need leave out only the foods that upset you. There are no reliable skin or blood tests as short cuts to discovering which foods you should avoid, and anyone with food intolerances has to work out his or her own long-term diet. However as a starting point, these are the diets we suggest for the different conditions:

Irritable bowel syndrome	Exclusion
Migraine	Exclusion
Asthma and rhinitis	Exclusion
Cow's milk sensitive enteropathy	Cow's milk-free
Coeliac disease	Gluten-free
Eczema	Cow's milk and egg-free Tartrazine and salicylate-free
Urticaria	Tartrazine and salicylate-free; if this is not successful, exclusion

Every recipe in this book is marked to show which of the diets it is suitable for, and on pages 24–32 we list substitute foods you can use by themselves or in the recipes. Here are some points about the different foods you may have to exclude, depending on the condition you have.

Cow's milk   Cow's milk is one of the commonest causes of food intolerances and it is taken in many forms besides just as a drink. A list of the foods containing it is given on page 33.

We mention 'milk substitute' in many recipes. This can be soya, goat's or sheep's milk. Dried cow's milk, skimmed, sterilized and UHT cow's milk are not suitable substitutes. Some evaporated cow's milks are said to be 'non-allergic' because they have been heated to a temperature high enough to destroy the proteins they contain. As food intolerance is not only an allergic problem, these milks are still likely to produce symptoms and so you should avoid them. The same is true of condensed milks.

Eggs   As well as not eating hens' eggs in any form, the egg-containing foods listed on page 34 have to be avoided. We don't recommend ducks' eggs as a substitute as they can contain infectious bacteria. Living on an egg-free diet may sound difficult, but there are plenty of egg-free baking recipes (and others where eggs would normally be used) in this book and they work very well.

Although there have been claims for quails' eggs, there is no scientific evidence that they are of any benefit to people with food intolerances.

Tartrazine and salicylates   Approximately one-fifth of our patients react to food additives such as preservatives and colourings. Tartrazine is a brilliant orange-yellow dye used in fruit squashes and many other foods – and even in some medicines. Some foods contain salicylates which are natural chemicals similar to aspirin. Foods containing salicylates which may also cause symptoms are:

apples	liquorice
bananas	peas
blueberries	plums and prunes
beer	red wine
cider	rhubarb
grapes	strawberries

Many other additives and preservatives can cause symptoms. In the UK, as a result of recent legislation, manufacturers are required to list all ingredients in foods, and this includes chemicals. You will find the system of code numbers for the different foods on page 113. This may help you discover exactly which additives are responsible for your problems (we have indicated those we allow on the exclusion diet).

Gluten and wheat   People with coeliac disease have to exclude entirely the protein called gluten found in wheat, rye and barley, and therefore all foods containing them as well. It is important to remember that a gluten-free diet and a wheat-free diet are not exactly the same. A lot of people have an intolerance to all wheat products and not only gluten. Some commercial gluten-free flours are prepared by removing the protein from wheat flour and replacing it by a protein from other sources. The wheat starch remains, so these products must be avoided by people testing for symptoms on the exclusion diet, and those who have wheat intolerance will find that foods made from these flours still cause symptoms.

The exclusion diet

This is the diet we use to discover our patients' food intolerances, and the one we recommend you follow to establish your own. We developed it by drawing up a list of the foods that upset the 122 people in our study (see page 19) who successfully controlled their symptoms. All the foods upsetting more than 20 per cent of the patients are excluded (for the full list, see page 29).

The advantage of this diet is that it is a healthy one of fresh and wholesome foods. People often lose weight and if they are rather fussy in their likes and dislikes, they may lose a little too much. To overcome this one slight problem, we give advice on quantities to eat during the trial period on page 36.

Following an exclusion diet

This will make a bigger impression on your lifestyle and your family's than any of the other food intolerance diets. Once you realize the strict exclusion will be for only two weeks, the idea shouldn't be too off-putting. Here is a plan for following your exclusion diet:

1. For three days before starting, record all the symptoms you have had, and when, to help judge the value of the diet later on.
2. For the first two weeks keep strictly to the diet outlined on page 29. Remember it is essential to continue for two weeks; all traces of offending foods eaten before the diet is begun must disappear from the body before symptoms clear, and so improvement is rarely seen in the first week. Don't give up; if you take a day off you will have wasted all your previous efforts, and will have to start again from the beginning.
3. During the first fortnight it is wise to exclude any foods besides those listed on page 29 that you may suspect have upset you; later on you will test and assess them properly.
4. It is better not to smoke.
5. During the second week you should eat as wide a variety of the 'allowed' foods as possible. This will help you notice any unusual food intolerances. Some foods allowed on the exclusion diet do upset a few people. They usually find out which these are in the second week of the diet and we explain how to deal with this in 7 below.
6. Throughout the second week keep an accurate diary of every food you eat, which symptoms you have, and when. Use a small notebook and allow a spread of two pages for each day (see the table on page 18).
7. You should find you steadily improve during the second week. Any unexpected setbacks at this time will probably have been caused by one of the foods eaten in the previous twenty-four hours. Compare the foods you recorded for

that day with the list in the table opposite. Any that upset 10 to 20 per cent of patients are the most likely to be the cause and if you have eaten one of these you should avoid it again until you have time to retest it.

8. If after two weeks your symptoms haven't improved, it is likely that food intolerance is not the cause of your problems. Go back to normal eating, and ask your doctor about trying other treatment.

Foods	Symptoms
Breakfast 8.00 a.m. Rice Krispies, apples, soya milk	
Mid-morning 11.15 a.m. Apple, camomile tea	Noon – diarrhoea × 1
Lunch 1.30 p.m. Chicken drumsticks, chick pea salad	2.30 p.m. – migraine
Afternoon 4.00 p.m. Water	started
Supper 8.00 p.m. Tomato juice, Bombay burgers, green salad, apple juice and oil dressing, Banana	

A day from a food diary

Reintroduction

You are no doubt feeling delighted by the improvement that the diet has brought. It is now highly likely that your symptoms can be controlled by diet. However, to find out exactly which foods are responsible still requires very careful planning. Continue to keep your diary throughout the reintroduction phase. The list below shows the order for reintroduction:

1. tap water
2. potatoes
3. cow's milk
4. yeast – take 3 brewer's yeast tablets or 2 tsp baker's yeast.
5. tea
6. rye – test rye crispbread and rye bread (check this is not a mixture of wheat and rye; only test rye bread if yeast was negative)
7. butter
8. onions
9. eggs
10. oats – test as porridge oats

Food	Percentage of patients affected	Food	Percentage of patients affected
Cereals		*Vegetables*	
wheat	60	onions	22
corn	44	potatoes	20
oats	34	cabbage	19
rye	30	sprouts	18
barley	24	peas	17
rice	15	carrots	15
		lettuce	15
		leeks	15
Dairy products		broccoli	14
milk	44	soya beans	13
cheese	39	spinach	13
eggs	26	mushrooms	12
butter	25	parsnips	12
yoghurt	24	tomatoes	11
		cauliflower	11
		celery	11
Fish		green beans	10
white fish	10	cucumber	10
shell fish	10	turnip/swede	10
smoked fish	7	marrow	8
		beetroot	8
		peppers	6
Meat		*Miscellaneous*	
beef	16	coffee	33
pork	14	tea	25
chicken	13	nuts	22
lamb	11	chocolate	22
turkey	8	preservatives	20
		yeast	20
		sugar cane	13
Fruit		sugar beet	12
citrus	24	alcohol	12
rhubarb	12	saccharin	9
apples	12	honey	2
banana	11		
pineapple	8		
pears	8		
strawberries	8		
grapes	7		
melon	5		
avocado pear	5		
raspberries	4		

Foods tested by patients attending our clinic

11. coffee – test coffee beans and instant coffee separately
12. chocolate – test plain chocolate
13. barley – pearl barley, added to soups and stews
14. citrus fruits
15. corn – test cornflour or corn on the cob (maize)
16. cow's cheese
17. white wine
18. shell fish
19. cow's yoghurt – test natural yoghurt, not flavoured
20. vinegar
21. wheat – test as wholemeal bread; white bread can be tested later; if yeast upsets you, test wheat as wheat-flakes
NB: Wheat produces its effects slowly so test for twice as long as other foods
22. nuts
23. preservatives – fruit squashes, tinned foods, monosodium glutamate (available from a delica-tessen), saccharin

How you begin reintroducing these foods depends on which condition you have. For migraine, irritable bowel syndrome, asthma and rhinitis we believe that one food should be reintroduced every two days. For eczema and urticaria a longer period of a week may be necessary. One method of testing is to use a rotating diet. We have not found this satisfactory as it quite often takes twenty-four to forty-eight hours for a reaction to a food to show, and on a rotating diet this leads to confusion about which food is responsible. Here are the rules to follow for reintroduction:

● If you have a reaction stop eating the food you are testing immediately or you may suffer severe symptoms; do not carry on testing new foods until you are completely well again. In any case, follow these instructions carefully and don't try to rush – the more haste, the less speed. The average reintroduction time for people we see is two months, with four visits to our clinic.

● The time it takes for symptoms to show also varies. Do not expect it always to be immediately after eating a food. Sometimes they appear so slowly that they are hardly noticeable. This is why it is so important to keep a diary – you can look back and see when you were last really well and this will help you spot the offending food.

● Eat plenty of the food you are testing – at least two good helpings a day. If after the last test day there are no ill-effects you may assume that the food is safe to eat in normal quantities, and use in cooking.

● Some foods (for example bread and wine) are made up of more than one ingredient. Test the ingredient concerned before trying the food: for example, test yeast before bread or wine; otherwise, if a reaction occurs, you will not know which ingredient caused it.

● It is wise to leave the testing of wheat until late in the reintroduction as this is the commonest cause of problems, and it is better to try it with a little experience under your belt.

● Flush out the chemicals in your system produced by the food reaction by drinking plenty of water. Some people find that adding a little bicarbonate of soda increases the effectiveness of this treatment. And don't forget, don't take pills to relieve any symptoms, for they confuse matters. Aspirin and paracetamol, for example, contain wheat and corn starches.

● Sometimes you may suspect that a food upsets you, but are not absolutely sure. Don't waste time testing and retesting one food; leave it out for two or three weeks and come back to it later when your diet is less restricted.

● At the end of the reintroduction you must go back and retest all foods you believe affect you. Some suspected reactions may have been coincidence and some food intolerances rapidly disappear. There is no point in avoiding a food unless you really have to.

● When you have finished your testing and identified all the foods which upset you, ask your doctor to arrange a visit to a dietitian to check that the diet you are planning to follow is properly nutritious.

● Unfortunately this reintroduction may not be final. Intolerances can change: operations, courses of antibiotics, virus infections and bouts of gastroenteritis are some of the reasons for this happening; it may be easy for you to identify a food that has brought back your symptoms but if you are unlucky you may have to take yourself right through the testing at any time in the future.

Will you be able to eat the upsetting foods again?
A reliable way to rid people of their intolerances has not yet been found. Several methods have been tried such as taking drops under the tongue, enzyme desensitization which involves putting drops on the skin, and various drugs, but they are still in the experimental stage and we have found all of them disappointing.

While the intolerance continues you will have to resign yourself to excluding the upsetting foods – as long as that seems preferable to suffering the symptoms.

However, many people find that after avoiding a food for some months it no longer upsets them, so recheck your food intolerances periodically – say every six months – and you may be pleasantly surprised. Coeliacs must of course always stick to their diet to avoid serious damage to the small intestine.

What should you do if you have many food intolerances?
If you are unlucky and find a large number of foods upset you, you should think seriously about whether it's worth trying to control your symptoms by diet, and you should certainly ask a dietitian to check the nutritional value of what you are eating and discuss other ways of coping with your symptoms with your doctor. If he or she feels that you can go on controlling your symptoms by diet rather than with drugs, it may help if you rotate your diet. We have found that when people can safely eat only a few foods, they eat so much of them that they may later get trouble with these foods as well. Rotating your diet means that you eat foods from each food family only every four or five days, so that you are not overexposed to any (food families are given on page 32).

Here is a suggested rotating diet; obviously you will have to adapt it according to your particular intolerances.

Day 1	Day 2	Day 3	Day 4
rice	potatoes	millet	buckwheat
poultry	lamb	fish	beef
carrots	tomatoes	broccoli	green beans
melon	pineapple	bananas	apples

Good nutrition on the exclusion diet

Energy   One of the main problems with the first stage of the exlusion diet is the provision of adequate energy or calories. As potatoes and bread are not allowed many people find it difficult to eat enough starchy carbohydrates to maintain their weight. Weight loss and hunger are very common when following this diet, and you should try to avoid them. Rice, millet and buckwheat with root vegetables such as parsnips, swede and turnips are good substitutes. As well as containing calories they give us protein, minerals and vitamins. We recommend the use of brown rice as this is more nutritious and contains more fibre than the highly refined white rice.

Recipes are also given for biscuits, cakes and puddings, which will help to fill you up. These should be used in moderation unless you find difficulty in keeping your weight steady. If you are overweight before starting the diet then do not use these sugary foods. Now is the time to lose those unhealthy extra pounds!

Fibre   With the exclusion of cereals such as wheat, rye and oats the fibre content of the diet will be lowered; fibre is of course very effective, not only in avoiding constipation, but many other bowel disorders. You should ensure your fibre intake is sufficient by eating plenty of brown rice, millet, buckwheat, fruit and vegetables. Pulses (such as kidney, soya and haricot beans) are particularly good sources of fibre. Aim to include at least 30g/1oz of fibre a day. To increase your fibre intake, soya and rice bran can be bought from a health food shop or chemist. If constipation becomes a problem despite these additions to the diet, buy a bulk laxative such as Isogel or Normacol from your chemist. These laxatives are made from the husks of plant seeds – a harmless form of roughage which has been used to help bowel conditions for many years in Eastern countries and very rarely upsets people with food intolerances.

Vitamins and minerals   As long as you eat widely on the exclusion diet you should avoid deficiencies. If, however, you are cow's milk intolerant and not using a milk substitute, calcium may be lacking and so supplements may be necessary. Calcium is available in other foods; alternatively you can take it in pills. Calcium lactate and gluconate are easily available from chemists.

   If you have become anaemic because of your condition, or you are intolerant of many iron-containing foods, you will need iron supplements. The best form is the ferrous sulphate mixture used for children, which has few ingredients. Your doctor can supply this.

   You should be very careful about taking extra vitamins, especially fat-soluble ones (A,D,E,K) as this can be dangerous, and the cult of 'megavitamins' has already led to people poisoning themselves in the USA. However, a small additional supplement of B vitamins often helps people on the exclusion diet, especially if they feel tired. Many vitamin pills are now produced free of wheat starch – check this with your doctor or chemist. A suitable daily vitamin B supplement would be:

Thiamine hydrochloride	150 mg
Riboflavine	15 mg
Nicotinamide	600 mg
Pyridoxine	100 mg
Ascorbic acid (vitamin C)	300 mg daily could be added to this

The best source of vitamin D is sunshine on the bare skin. Get out and about as often as you can, especially on sunny days. A holiday in the sun is of tremendous benefit.

Enjoying your food

If you find that you have food intolerances you cannot expect your diet to be just the same as ever, any more than you expect the food to be the same abroad as at home. You have to be willing to experiment a little and get used to new tastes and textures. Most people's eating habits have to fit in with their families' and friends', so we have tried to include dishes that they will enjoy too. Old favourites such as Sunday roast lunches are fine, and can be easily adapted to suit your diet. There are substitutes for all the common ingredients such as wheat products and cow's milk, and we show here how you can use them in your cooking.

Grains and flours

The gluten in flours used for baking is elastic and holds air. This is why a strong (high-gluten) wheat flour is ideal for breadmaking. Grains suitable for coeliacs or people with wheat intolerance are less likely to rise and great patience is needed to master the skills of breadmaking with gluten-free flours (we give advice on page 88).

Most of the flours listed are obtainable from wholefood or health food shops, or may be milled from the grains in a powerful domestic blender.

Arrowroot is a starchy root with the consistency of cornflour. It is almost pure starch, providing little besides carbohydrate and is most useful as a thickening agent for gravies and sauces.

Another exotic thickener is *kuzu* from Japan.

Buckwheat is confusingly named as it comes from plants of the same family as dock leaves and so is all right for people with wheat intolerance. It is available in health food shops. The flour, which has a strong and distinctive flavour, has an egg-like binding capacity which makes it very good in batters. It contains some protein and is rich in B vitamins. Some buckwheat products (for example, spaghetti) are sold ready-made. Read the labels with special care as many also contain wheat flour.

Carob flour is ground from the pod of the locust tree and has a strong chocolate taste. As well as being high in pectin, it contains appreciable amounts of proteins, carbohydrates, calcium and phosphorus. It is an invaluable alternative to chocolate for flavouring cakes and drinks.

Chestnut flour is derived from the sweet chestnut. It does have a distinctive flavour and is rather heavy, but can be used for baking cakes and biscuits (for example, shortbread, scones, fruit crumbles or crisps).

Gram flour is made from ground pulses. It is widely used in Indian breads and batters and, like soya flour, is high in protein, vitamins and minerals. It has a strong flavour and will go bitter if kept too long.

Maize meal (also known as corn meal) is a good thickening agent. It may be used in baking cakes, biscuits and bread, or for the

Italian dish, *polenta* (similar to porridge but eaten with savoury food).

Millet, like rice, is a member of the grass family, but both are distant enough relatives of wheat to be safe for many people with wheat intolerance. It has good nutritional value, providing B vitamins, minerals and proteins. Millet is available as a grain, a flake or a flour. It can be used in a variety of sweet and savoury dishes as it is filling and pleasant-tasting.

Potato flour, sometimes called *fécule* or *farina*, is an excellent thickening agent and useful for baking. It is a pure starch with little flavour of its own. (NB Instant mashed potato contains chemical additives and is not a substitute for pure potato flour.)

Rice. Brown rice is preferable to white as it contains many vitamins (especially group B) as well as minerals and fibre.

Rice flour, rice flakes and ground rice can be used in baking biscuits and making puddings. Rice flour is best mixed with other flours as it has a strong flavour.

Sago flour is like rice flour in texture but comes from the trunk of the palm tree. It is good for puddings, and thickening stews, and has no strong flavour.

Soya flour is made from ground soya beans. It is an excellent source of protein, fat and B vitamins. It has a strong flavour and is best used in combination with other dishes, where it increases the protein value.

Tapioca comes from the root of a tropical plant (cassava). Like sago it is almost pure starch. It is used by itself to make a pudding, but is also handy for thickening soups and stews.

Cooking grains

Brown rice   Wash and drain the rice. Allow twice the volume of cooking water to rice. Bring the water to the boil, add rice and ½ to 1 tsp salt, depending on quantity being cooked. Turn heat down, cover and simmer for about 40 minutes until tender and the water is absorbed. Do not stir the rice while it is cooking as this breaks up the grains. Fluff with a fork when ready.

Buckwheat   This grain can be bought either roasted or unroasted, the roasted being rather stronger in flavour. The type you choose depends on your preference. Put the buckwheat into twice its volume of cold salted water, bring to the boil and simmer until all the moisture has been absorbed and the buckwheat is soft (about 15 minutes). Unroasted buckwheat takes slightly longer to cook than roasted. Do not stir while cooking.

Millet   Cook as for buckwheat. In some savoury dishes millet can be dry roasted in the pan first to enhance the flavour.

Dairy products

Cheese   A large number of excellent cheeses made from goat's or ewe's milk are available. These are listed on page 31. There is also a cheese made from soya milk.

Cooking fats   As a cow's milk product, butter is not allowed. In most recipes we have used Tomor margarine as it is easily available in large supermarkets and health food stores, and milk-free. Those in the UK who have difficulty finding a stockist should contact the makers: Van den Berghs and Jurgens Ltd, Sussex House, Burgess Hill, West Sussex, RH15 9AW. In North America and Australia, similar margarines made entirely from vegetable products can be used.

Lard is derived from animal fats and so is unlikely to cause problems to most people with milk intolerance. Those who prefer to cook with unsaturated fats may use oils such as safflower or sunflower. Commercial 'vegetable oil' is a blend and usually contains maize (or corn) oil.

Ewe's milk is not a widely available product but you may find it in some country localities. It is certainly worth trying, although we have no personal experience of its use. We do have reports that sheep's milk yoghurt is very palatable. For a list of UK suppliers of dairy products from sheep, contact Mrs Olivia Mills, Weald Wood Farm, Alresford, Hampshire.

Goat's milk is widely available from health food stores, but you need to be reassured about its source. Goat's milk is not pasteurized, and sometimes carries salmonella, but very rarely TB or brucellosis. Home pasteurization is impractical, but boiling the milk is useful. Goat's milk can be stored in the refrigerator or deep frozen (many people prefer to drink it chilled). In the UK dried goat's milk is available by mail order from: Welsh Goats Ltd, Unit 1, Industrial Estate, Tregaron, Dyfed SY23 5LE Wales.

The value of goat's milk is limited. People whose asthma, hayfever or eczema are caused by cow's milk and who have switched to goat's milk often find that they then become intolerant to this. Similarly, some people with irritable bowel syndrome have found goat's milk only a temporary help.

Soya milk is made from soya beans and may be obtained from wholefood shops (Plamil, Itona and Granose are a few of the brands). Unopened it keeps without refrigeration but should be kept in the refrigerator for no more than three days after opening. Commercially produced soya milk doesn't have a strong flavour and it can be used in cooking as an alternative to cow's milk. Some brands contain cane sugar, sea salt and sunflower oil to enhance the flavour. You can make your own soya milk from soya flour:

Soya milk

Makes approximately 1½ pints

150 g/5 oz soya flour
Vanilla pod, honey or concentrated apple juice (optional)

Mix flour with 1 1/2 pints water in a saucepan. Bring slowly to the boil, stirring all the time. (Caution! This mixture quickly froths over like cow's milk when boiling.) Reduce the heat and simmer for 20 minutes, stirring frequently.

The milk can be flavoured with honey, apple juice or vanilla pod. Add apple juice when the milk has cooled, otherwise it curdles.

Use as a milk substitute. Store in a refrigerator as it ferments when exposed to heat.

Savoury flavourings

Miso is a fermented mixture of cereal grains, soya beans, water and salt. The form containing rice will be suitable for many with food intolerance, but be careful not to confuse this with other varieties containing wheat or barley. Miso is rich in protein, minerals and vitamins, including vitamin B_{12}. It has a thick, pasty consistency and is thinned with water (but not boiling as this curdles it) to be used as a stock base in soups, stews, sauces and gravies.

Tahini   This is made from sesame seeds crushed and blended with oil. It is useful for making sauces and in the dip, hummus. For people who can't tolerate lemon, an added amount of garlic and parsley makes an excellent alternative. Tahini can also be included in salad dressing or used as a sandwich spread.

Drinks

Hot carob-flavoured soya milk is relaxing at bedtime (use the carob flour like cocoa powder). Earlier in the day, pineapple juice is refreshing. Herbal teas, matté and chicory are handy. Some teas come in individual tea-bags which are useful to take to work. Ground chicory can be brewed in the same way as ground coffee. Try apple juice, or grape and apple juice mix, with ice and a sprig of mint, or tomato juice with a touch of paprika. These are sophisticated enough to drink in the early evening, and you can become quite a connoisseur of mineral water with your dinner.

Some mineral waters are still, some naturally sparkling and some artificially carbonated and described as sparkling. Many supermarket own brands fall into this category, and are very gassy. Perrier has a small mineral content and strong effervescence. Badiot from St Galmer in the Loire produces a softly sparkling water with medium mineral content. Vichy-Celestin is another natural sparkler: it has a higher mineral content than Badiot. A particularly flavoured mineral water with a very high mineral content is St-Yorre, which sparkles and has a strong salty alkaline taste. Delicious still waters abound in Britain: Malvern is the most famous, but water from springs in Orchil in the Highlands, from Shropshire and from Wales are also easily available.

Shopping: foods to buy and foods to avoid

On the following pages we list some of the less well-known fresh fruits and vegetables normally acceptable to people with food intolerances, and suggest ways of cooking them as they introduce as much variety as possible into a restricted diet. We also list the foods, especially processed foods, that you should avoid, at least on the first part of the exclusion diet. Armed with this information, you should not find shopping for your special diet too confusing or off-putting. (For food labelling, see the Appendix on page 113.)

Always buy fresh or frozen foods. Ingredients in tinned and packet foods should be checked for food additives, which must be avoided as far as possible. The table opposite is a general guide to categories of allowed and not-allowed foods during the first two weeks of the exclusion diet. For more detailed information on the latter, see pages 33–6. We suggest here some unusual foods to vary your diet.

Vegetables

Celeriac has a mild celery flavour. Add chopped to soups or casseroles or cook and serve puréed with game. Very good grated raw in salads. Another way of serving is to peel, shred and blanch the celeriac and mix with mayonnaise, garlic and mustard.

Fennel has a crunchy texture with a mild aniseed flavour. Serve raw, shredded in salads or boil until tender and serve with white sauce. Excellent with fish. The feathery leaves can be used to flavour salads.

Mange-tout (sugar peas) have a sweet and crisp flavour. Top and tail then boil for 1–2 minutes. Serve tossed in vegetable margarine. Can also be served raw, finely sliced in salads.

Okra (ladies' fingers) are soft and have a syrupy texture. Top each pod and boil for five minutes. Delicious with curries or a tomato sauce.

Plantain tastes like banana but is less sweet. It is always eaten cooked. Peel, boil and mash, or bake whole in its skin.

Foods for the exclusion diet

	Not allowed	Allowed
Meat	preserved meats, bacon, sausages	all other meats
Fish	smoked fish, shell fish	white fish
Vegetables	potatoes, onions, sweetcorn	all other vegetables, salads, pulses, swede and parsnip
Fruit	citrus fruit, eg, oranges, grapefruit	all other fruit, eg, apples, bananas, pears
Cereals	wheat (see page 34), oats, barley, rye, corn (see page 35)	rice, ground rice, rice flakes, rice flour, sago, Rice Krispies, tapioca, millet, buckwheat, rice cakes
Cooking oils	corn oil, vegetable oil	sunflower oil, soya oil, safflower oil, olive oil
Dairy products	cow's milk (see page 33), butter, most margarines, cow's milk, yoghurt and cheese, eggs	goat's milk, soya milk, sheep's milk, Tomor margarine, goat's and sheep's milk yoghurt and cheese, soya cheese
Beverages	tea, coffee – beans, instant and decaffeinated, fruit squashes, orange juice, grapefruit juice, alcohol, tap water	herbal teas, eg, camomile, fresh fruit juices, eg, apple, pineapple, tomato juice, mineral, distilled or de-ionized water
Miscellaneous	chocolates, yeast (see page 35), preservatives (see page 16)	carob, sea salt, herbs, spices; in moderation: sugar, honey

NB Some fruits, especially overripe ones, contain small amounts of yeast but the quantities rarely cause any problems.

Pumpkin has a juicy, delicate flavour. Remove the skin, pith and seeds. Cut flesh into small chunks and boil for ten minutes, or steam. Serve with cheese sauce. Can also be used in curries, soups or sweet puddings.

Salsify has a flavour similar to Jerusalem artichokes. Peel and boil in salted water with a few drops of lemon juice (if allowed) until tender. Cut into pieces and serve with melted vegetable margarine, lemon juice and herbs, or with a cheese sauce. Alternatively chop and fry in margarine until deep golden brown and serve with a squeeze of lemon juice.

Suggestions for vegetable combinations

First vegetable	How cooked	Second vegetable	How cooked	Combine and serve
brussels sprouts	boiled in salted water	sweet chestnuts	peeled and fried in Tomor for 2 minutes	add sprouts to Tomor and nut mixture, stir and fry a further few minutes
Carrot, grated	fried	chopped chicory heads, chopped bean sprouts	fried for the last 5 minutes	Stir in apple juice for last minute of frying and season
celery	sticks, 4 cm/1½ in long, ½ cm/¼ in wide, lightly boiled	walnut pieces	fried in Tomor	add celery to Tomor and nut mixture, stir and fry a further few minutes
courgette	sliced and simmered with mint and peas for 5–6 minutes	peas	simmered with mint and courgette	toss in melted Tomor with chopped chives
french beans	fried in Tomor with mixed herbs	crisp lettuce	added to beans for last 5 minutes	hot, immediately
leeks, washed and cut into 3 cm/1 in long pieces	boiled in salted water	skinned and chopped tomatoes	fried in oil with slices of garlic	pour tomatoes over chopped leeks, garnish with chopped parsley
red cabbage	shredded and boiled 5–10 minutes with a few caraway seeds	red pepper	fried in oil for 1 minute with cabbage	hot, immediately
runner beans	boiled in salted water	finely chopped celery, skinned, chopped tomatoes	fried in garlic and oil	stir yoghurt into cooked celery and tomato mixture, add concentrated tomato purée; serve on beans garnished with chopped parsley
spinach	boiled in very little salted water	celery	chopped and fried in oil	season and stir spinach into celery, fry a further few minutes
spinach	boiled in very little lightly salted water	goat's yoghurt	stir in crushed garlic and season	mix together well and serve hot

Sweet potatoes can be substituted for potatoes. They have a similar flavour to Jerusalem artichokes. Can be boiled, baked or steamed. If boiled add a little lemon juice to the water to prevent discolouring (provided it is allowed). Very good mashed and flavoured with cinnamon, nutmeg or orange.

Water chestnuts have a delicate, juicy flavour, with a crisp nutty texture. Wash and peel carefully. Add raw to salads, toast or stir fry.

Yams Substitute for potatoes. They have a faint nutty flavour. Cook and serve as for sweet potatoes.

Fruits

Guava has a firm milky texture and a faint strawberry flavour. Peel and eat alone or with fruit salad. Use for sorbets and for making jam.

Kiwi fruit (Chinese gooseberries) have a delicious sharp taste. Peel and slice thinly into fruit or vegetable salads.

Lychees have the texture of a grape. Peel and eat alone.

Mango has a sweet and slightly gingery flavour. Remove skin and stone. Use in fruit salads, ice cream, sorbets and for making chutneys.

Passion fruit has a sweet, seedy pulp. Remove top and scoop out flesh. Eat alone or add to fruit salads.

Pawpaw is similar to a melon, with a faint scented flavour. Slice in half, remove black seeds and eat raw, sprinkled with lemon juice if allowed.

Physalis is a tart citrus berry. Remove husk, eat raw or use in pies or tarts.

Sharon fruit is a seedless persimmon tasting like a sweet peach. Slice into fruit salads or blend with ice cream.

French cheeses made with sheep's or goat's milk
Cheeses marked with an asterisk are the most easily obtainable. The others are likely to be found only in their own area of production.

Cheese	Type of milk
Arnéguy	sheep's
Asco	goat's
Bougon*	goat's
Bouton-de-Culotte	goat's
Chabichou*	goat's
Chevrotin*	goat's

Cheese	Type of milk
Chevrotin persillé des Aravis*	goat's
Crottin de Chavignol*	goat's
Iraty	sheep's
Laruns	sheep's
Levroux	goat's
Macon	goat's
Pélardon	goat's
Picodon	goat's
Pouligny-Saint-Pierre	goat's
Pyramide*	goat's
Roquefort*	sheep's
Ruffec	goat's
Saint-Foy	goat's
Saint-Maixent	goat's
Saint-Maure	goat's
Sancerre	goat's
Selle-sur-Cher	goat's
Tome d'Arles*	sheep's
Valençay	goat's

Food families

It is useful to know which family particular foods belong to since intolerance to one may mean that other members of the group cause symptoms.

Plants

Caricaceae: pawpaw

Chenopodiaceae: beetroot, spinach, sugar beet

Compositae: artichokes (globe and Jerusalem), camomile, chicory, endive, lettuce, safflower, salsify, sunflower, tarragon

Convolvulaceae: sweet potato

Cruciferae: Brussels sprouts, broccoli, cabbage, cauliflower, Chinese cabbage, horseradish, kale, kohl rabi, mustard, rape, swede, turnip, watercress

Cucurbitaceae: cucumber, courgette, marrow, melon, pumpkin

Cycadaceae: sago

Dioscoreaceae: yam

Ebenaceae: persimmon

Ericaceae: bilberry, blueberry, cranberry

Euphorbiaceae: cassava, tapioca

Fungi: mushrooms

Gramineae: barley, corn, millet, oats, rice, rye, sugar cane, wheat

Labiatae: balm, basil, mint, marjoram, oregano, peppermint, rosemary, sage

Leguminosae: dry beans, green beans, lentils, liquorice, peas, peanuts

Liliaceae: asparagus, chives, garlic, leek, onion

Malvaceae: okra
Marantaceae: arrowroot
Moraceae: mulberry
Musaceae: banana, plantain
Myrtaceae: guava
Onagraceae: water chestnut
Palmae: coconut, dates
Passifloraceae: passion fruit
Polygonaceae: buckwheat, rhubarb
Rosaceae: apple, apricot, blackberry, cherry, loganberry, nectarine, peach, pear, plum, prune, raspberry, strawberry,
Rubiaceae: coffee
Rutaceae: grapefruit, lemon, lime, mandarin, orange, tangerine
Saxifragaceae: gooseberry, black and red currants
Solanaceae: aubergine, cayenne, paprika, pepper, potato, physalis, tobacco, tomato
Theaceae: tea
Umbelliferae: angelica, caraway, carrots, celeriac, celery, coriander, dill, fennel, parsley, parsnips, samphire,
Vitaceae: grape, vine

Animal
Dairy products: butter, cheese, milk, yoghurt
Crustaceans: crab, crayfish, lobster, prawn, shrimp
Molluscs: clam, mussel, oyster, scallop, snail, squid

Food containing cow's milk and cow's milk products
Milk is used in a variety of manufactured products. Check all labels on bought foods and if the following items are contained do not use that product: milk, butter, margarine, cream, cheese, yoghurt, skimmed milk powder, non-fat milk solids, caseinates, whey, lactalbumin, lactose.
The foods listed below are likely to contain milk and/or milk products, so always check the list of ingredients:

biscuits
bread, bread mixes
breakfast cereals
cakes, cake mixes
gravy mixes
malted milk drinks, eg, Horlicks, Ovaltine, Bournvita
puddings and mixes, ice cream, junket, custards
ready meals: fish, meat, rice and pasta dishes
sauces, cream soups
sausages
sweets, eg, milk chocolate, fudge, toffee
vegetables canned in sauce

Foods containing eggs

Foods containing egg yolk, egg white, and lecithin should be avoided. The following may contain eggs:

baked foods – cakes, biscuits, pastry and batter
egg noodles and pasta
lemon curd
malted milk drink, eg, Bournvita
mayonnaise
puddings and mixes
soups

Foods containing wheat

Wheat is present in the following products. Check all labels on manufactured foods. If wheat, wheat starch, edible starch, cereal filler, cereal binder or cereal protein are listed in the ingredients do not use that product. Foods marked with an asterisk may or may not contain wheat.

Beverages: cocoa,* drinking chocolate,* coffee essence,* milk shake flavourings,* Horlicks, Ovaltine,*
Biscuits: homemade and bought
Bread: including white, wholemeal, wholewheat, granary breads, rye bread,* slimming bread, Energen rolls
Breakfast cereals, eg, Shredded Wheat, Puffed Wheat, All-Bran, Weetabix, muesli,* Bemax, Grapenuts, baby cereals*
Cakes: including homemade and bought cakes, cake mixes and scones
Dairy products and fats: cheese spreads,* processed cheese,* packet suet*
Fish: tinned,* fish paste,* fish cooked in batter, breadcrumbs or a sauce
Flours and cereals: ordinary wheat flours, bran, wheatgerm, semolina, pasta, noodles
Fruit: pie fillings*
Meat: tinned,* ready meals,* pies, sausage rolls, meat paste,* pâté,* sausages*
Pastry: homemade, bought, mixes and frozen
Puddings: packet puddings, dessert mixes,* ice cream,* mousses,* custard powder*
Soups: tinned and packets
Vegetables: tinned in sauces, eg, baked beans,* tinned vegetable salad,* instant potato powder*
Miscellaneous: stuffings, savoury spreads,* mayonnaise,* curry powder,* mustard,* chutney,* mincemeat,* peanut butter,*

lemon curd,* lemon cheese,* sweets and chocolates,* baking powder,* gravy browning,* stock cubes,* soy sauce,* pepper compounds, packet seasonings

Foods containing yeast

The following products can, and frequently do, contain yeast in one form or another.

Bread: any kind of bread, except soda bread
Bread sauce, bread pudding, stuffings made with breadcrumbs, breadcrumb coatings on, eg, fish fingers, fish cakes, potato croquettes
Buns made with yeast eg, teacakes, rolls, crumpets, doughnuts
Cheese, yoghurt, buttermilk, soured cream, synthetic cream
Cream crackers, Twiglets
Fermented beverages, eg, wine, beer, cider
Fruit juice (home squeezed citrus fruits are yeast-free)
Yeast extract, Bovril, most stock cubes and gravy browning, tinned and packet soups
Grapes, sultanas, currants, plums, dates, prunes and products containing these, eg, fruit cake, mincemeat, muesli, raisin bran
Malted milk drinks, eg, Ovaltine, Horlicks
Meat products containing bread, eg, sausages, meat loaf, beefburgers
Overripe fruit
Pizza
Puddings made with bread, eg, apple charlotte, summer pudding
Vinegar and pickled foods, eg, pickled onions, pickled beetroot, sauces containing vinegar, eg, tomato ketchup, salad dressing, mayonnaise
Vitamin products: most B vitamin products contain yeast

Foods containing corn

The products listed can and frequently do contain corn in one form or another, as corn starch, oil, syrup or cornmeal. Edible starch, food starch, maize oil, glucose syrup, vegetable oil and dextrose are also usually derived from corn. Always check the label of manufactured products. Products marked with an asterisk may or may not contain corn.

Baking mixtures for cakes and biscuits*
Baking powders*
Bleached white flour
Bottled sauces – many contain food starch or syrup*
Cakes and biscuits*
Canned foods, eg, soups, puddings, baked beans*

Cornflakes
Cornflour
Custard powder
Gravy browning
Ices, ice creams*
Instant puddings*
Instant teas, eg, lemon tea mix contains dextrose
Jams, jellies*
Margarine and vegetable oils containing corn oil
Peanut butter*
Polenta
Popcorn
Salad dressings*
Sweets – may be sweetened with corn syrup, eg, sherbets, marshmallows
Tortillas

Sample menus

These are rough guides to the amount of food which should be eaten when following the first stage of the exclusion diet. They are worked out for men and women of ideal weight. If you are over-weight, cut down on both fats and sugars. Do not fry foods, use only a scraping of vegetable margarine on biscuits and do not use it on vegetables. Do not eat sugary foods such as cakes and puddings. It is important, however, to maintain a sufficient fibre intake, so eat plenty of starchy foods high in fibre, for example, brown rice, buckwheat, fruits and vegetables.

If you are underweight, try having snacks between meals. Recipes are given for sweet and savoury biscuits and cakes which you may find useful. Increase the amount of milk substitute to 600 ml/1 pt a day. Milky drinks such as carob milk are very tasty. If your appetite is good you can also have larger main meals. More meat, fish, vegetables and rice can be taken. A pudding will also help provide extra calories.

Meal plan for adults of ideal weight
The foods and quantities given below can be eaten by anyone using this book. Extra recommendations for men are given in brackets.

Daily: 275–425 ml/½–¾ pt milk substitute [425 ml/¾ pt]

Breakfast
Fruit juice
30 g/1 oz Rice Krispies with milk substitute
2 buckwheat and rice crackers with Tomor margarine [4]
2 portions fruit, eg, apple, banana

Lunch
Fruit juice
100 g/3½ oz meat or 150 g/5 oz fish
large helping vegetables or salad
90 g/3 oz brown rice, buckwheat or millet [120 g/4 oz]
2 portions fruit [2 crackers with Tomor margarine in addition]

Supper
Fruit juice
100 g/3½ oz meat or 150 g/5 oz fish
large helping vegetables or salad
90 g/3 oz brown rice, buckwheat or millet [120 g/4 oz]
Pudding, eg, milk pudding made with sago

Bedtime
Fruit juice
2 portions fruit

Suggested menus: Exclusion diet

Breakfast
Apple juice
Muesli and milk substitute
Buckwheat and rice crackers with Tomor margarine

Lunch
Spiced apple juice
Stuffed tomatoes
Green salad
Anytime-of-year fruit salad with sheep's yogurt

Supper
Fruit cocktail
Celeriac soup
Rosemary and garlic lamb
Millet
Carrots
Apricot mould

Bedtime
Carob milk drink

Wheat-free diet

Breakfast
Fruit juice
Millet flake granola and milk
Buckwheat brown bread and butter with marmalade

Lunch
Pizza

Mixed salad
Dried fruit compote

Supper
Melon and grape savoury starter
Balkan chops
Green beans
Baked potatoes
Fruit flan

Milk-free diet

Breakfast
Fruit juice
Millet flake granola with milk substitute
Toast, Tomor, marmalade

Lunch
Savoury buckwheat pancakes
Mixed salad
Baked bananas and nut cream

Supper
Chestnut soup and wholemeal rolls
Turkey with apple and cherries
Carrots
Potatoes
Summer fruit dessert

Egg-free diet

Breakfast
Fruit juice
Muesli and milk
Grilled bacon and tomato
Wholemeal bread, butter and yeast extract

Lunch
Chicken Waldorf
Savoury rice
Stuffed baked apples

Supper
Four-meat pâté with white toast
Crispy coated fish
Creamed spinach
Potatoes
Peach condé

THE RECIPES

All the recipes in this book are as far as possible free from artificial colourings, flavourings and preservatives. They are also free from gluten (wheat, rye and barley), other wheat, corn, oats and cow's milk. If you simply want to exclude one or more of these from your diet you may choose any recipe you wish. If you are following the first stage of the exclusion diet or are excluding eggs you should select only those appropriately marked. If other foods are to be excluded you will need to examine the list of ingredients in each recipe carefully to see whether it is suitable for your diet.

Where you are advised to use a milk substitute, use any that is suitable for you, such as goat's, sheep's or soya milk.

Symbols
The symbols used in this book for the specials diets are:

★	exclusion
W	wheat-free
M	milk-free
E	egg-free

Measurements
The measurements are given in both metric and imperial units. Use one system only; do not combine them.

Where spoonfuls are referred to, level spoons are meant unless otherwise stated.

1 tsp (teaspoon) = 5 ml
1 tbsp (tablespoon) = 15 ml

To ensure success, check the size of the spoons you are using. Australian users should remember that as their tablespoon has been converted to 20 ml, and is therefore larger than the tablespoon measurements used in the recipes in this book, they should use 3 × 5 ml tsp where instructed to use 1 × 15 ml tbsp.

BREAKFASTS

Muesli

Serves 6

170 g/6 oz buckwheat or millet
225 g/8 oz brown rice

120 g/4 oz dried fruit (eg, apricots,
peaches, raisins)
2 tbsp honey if desired

Cook the buckwheat, millet or rice according to instructions (see page 25). Cool. Mix with chopped dried fruit. Honey can be added to sweeten the muesli.
Serve with milk substitute

Millet flake granola

Makes 565 g/1¼ lb granola

225 g/8 oz millet flakes
120 g/4 oz nuts (mixed flaked almonds,
chopped hazelnuts)

8 tbsp honey
1 tbsp oil
120 g/4 oz raisins

Preheat oven to 180 °C/350 °F/gas 4.
Mix millet·flakes, nuts, honey and oil together. Spread mixture thinly over 2 baking sheets.
Bake for 30 minutes, turning occasionally so that the millet is evenly and lightly browned.
Cool the crumble. Mix in the raisins.
Store in a sealed jar for up to 1 month.
Serve as a breakfast cereal with milk or on top of yoghurt or fruit as a dessert.

Buckwheat breakfast

Serves 4

4 buckwheat pancakes (see page 45)   sugar, salt, pepper, mixed herbs
tomatoes, sliced

Cook pancakes according to instructions.
Grill tomato slices lightly sprinkled with sugar, salt, pepper and mixed herbs for 1–2 minutes until just cooked.
Place on pancakes and serve.

Milkshake (*top*, see page 46), Millet flake granola (*centre*), Buckwheat breakfast (*bottom*) OVERLEAF: Melon and grape savoury starter (*top left*, see page 48), Fruit cocktail (*top right*, see page 47), Sophisticated swiss roll (*bottom left*, see page 49), Cocktail nibbles (*bottom right*, see page 48)

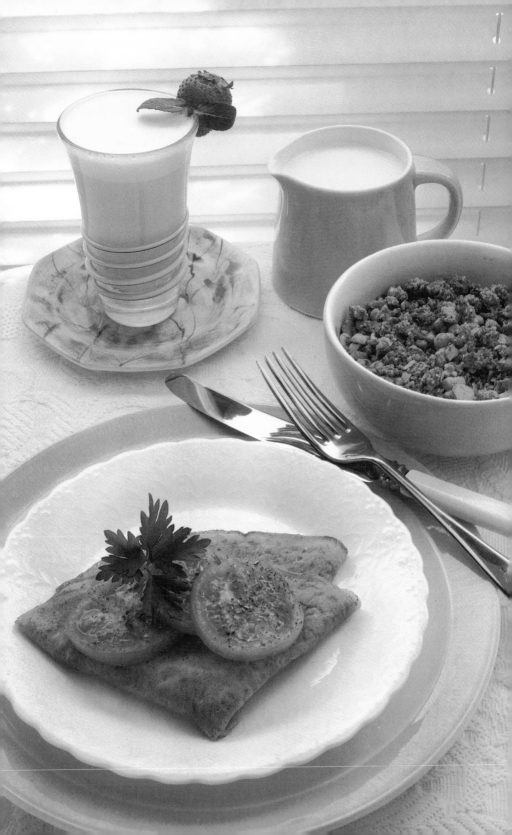

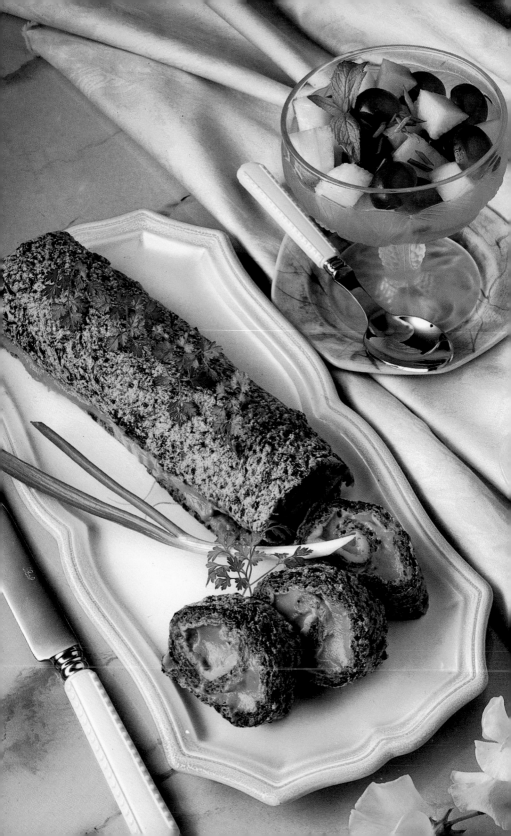

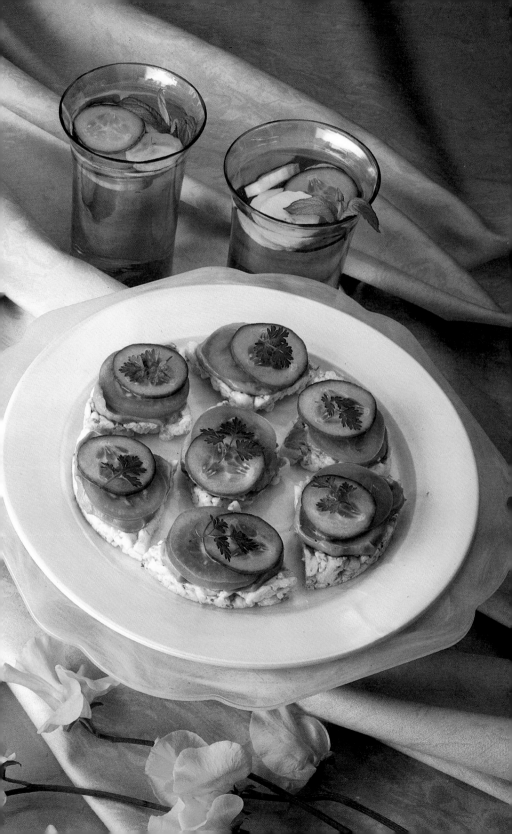

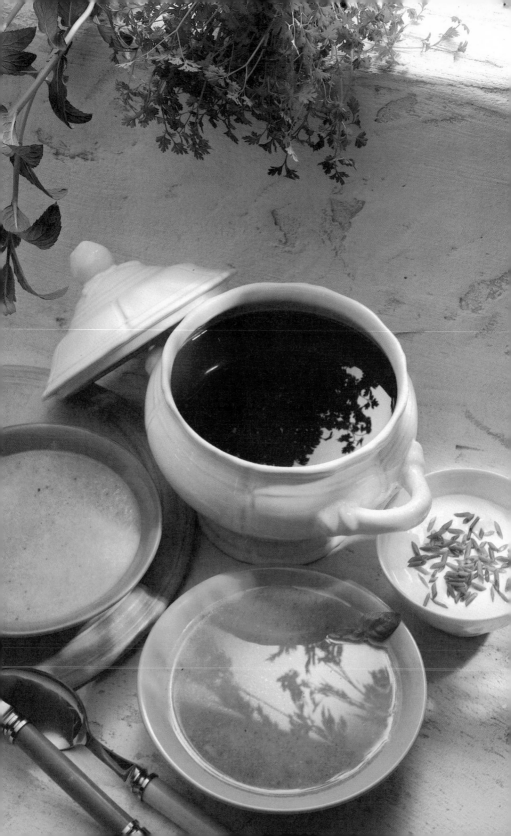

Hot fruity breakfast

Serves 1

*30 g/1 oz lightly crushed millet,
  toasted*
120 ml/4 fl oz milk substitute

*stewed fruit (gooseberries are good,
  fresh or bottled)*
golden syrup (optional)

Mix the millet and milk in a pan, bring gently to the boil and simmer for 5 minutes, stirring occasionally.

Put in serving bowl, stir in 1–2 tbsp stewed fruit, and serve with extra milk substitute or a luxurious blob of golden syrup.

Buckwheat pancakes

Serves 4

(1)

60 g/2 oz buckwheat flour
60 g/2 oz rice flour
*1 tbsp Tomor margarine, melted in a
  saucepan, or 1 tbsp of oil*

⅛ tsp sea salt
*1 tsp commercial wheat-free baking
  powder (see page 89)*
300 ml/½ pint milk substitute

Sift the flours and salt together. Mix with melted margarine or oil and milk substitute and beat well. Leave to stand for 30 minutes before using. Just before using stir in the baking powder.

To make the pancakes, put about ⅔ tbsp oil into a frying pan and heat until just beginning to smoke. Quickly pour in enough batter to coat the base of the pan thinly and tilt the pan to make sure that the batter runs evenly all over. Let the pancake set and brown underneath, then turn it gently with a broad bladed knife – do not toss the pancake – and brown it on the other side.

Serve with savoury or sweet fillings.

(2)   W M

60 g/2 oz buckwheat flour
60 g/2 oz rice flour
⅛ tsp salt

1 egg
300 ml/½ pint milk substitute

Sift flour and salt together. Mix with egg and milk, beat well. Leave to stand for 30 minutes before using. Cook as above.

Bortsch with yoghurt (*top*, see page 49), Chestnut soup (*centre*, see page 50), Tomato and courgette soup (*bottom*, see page 52)

BEVERAGES

Milk shake ⊞ Ⓦ Ⓜ Ⓔ

Serves 4   See photograph, page 41

400 ml/⅔ pint milk substitute   *1 banana*
400 ml/⅔ pint fruit juice

Blend together in a liquidizer, or mash banana and whip with milk and fruit juice. Chill before serving.

Alternatives This is very refreshing made with pineapple juice.
    Soft fruits such as strawberries, and stewed blackcurrants could be substituted for the fruit juice and banana in the recipe.

Carob milk drink ⊞ Ⓦ Ⓜ Ⓔ

Serves 2

1 tsp honey   *300 ml/½ pint milk substitute*
1 tbsp carob flour

Whip together or blend in a liquidizer. Chill, or serve hot.

Minty yoghurt ⊞ Ⓦ Ⓜ Ⓔ

Serves 2

300 ml/½ pint goat's or ewe's yoghurt
1 tbsp fresh chopped mint

Whip or blend together in a liquidizer the yoghurt, mint and up to 120 ml/4 fl oz water, depending on thickness of the yoghurt. Chill.
    Very good served with Indian food.

Pineapple yoghurt drink ⊞ Ⓦ Ⓜ Ⓔ

Serves 2

200 ml/7 fl oz goat's or ewe's yoghurt   *2 tsp sugar (optional)*
180 ml/6 fl oz pineapple juice

Whip together or blend in a liquidizer. Chill before serving.

Fruit cocktail   ⊠ ☐W ☐M ☐E

Serves 4

See photograph, page 42

600 ml/1 pint apple juice
4 tbsp mixed chopped fruit, eg, peach,
  banana, cucumber

Mix together and chill before serving.

Spiced apple juice   ⊠ ☐W ☐M ☐E

Serves 4

400 ml/⅔ pint apple juice   *⅛ tsp ginger*
6 cloves   *⅛ tsp nutmeg*
⅛ tsp cinnamon   *2 tsp honey (optional)*

Put all ingredients into a saucepan with 200 ml/⅓ pint water. Heat but do not boil. Allow the spices to infuse for a few minutes. Strain before serving.
   Makes a warming winter drink.

Coconut milk   ⊠ ☐W ☐M ☐E

Makes 600 ml/1 pint

85 g/3 oz desiccated coconut   *1 tbsp honey*

Add coconut to 300 ml/½ pint water and bring to simmering point slowly. Remove from heat, cool and liquidize until smooth. Strain through a fine sieve, pressing out as much of the liquid as possible. Return coconut to saucepan and repeat using 300 ml/½ pint water; simmer, liquidize and sieve. Mix both batches of milk with the honey. Chill and store in a refrigerator. Stir before serving.
   Can be used as a drink or in puddings or on cereals.

STARTERS AND SOUPS

Cocktail nibbles

1 avocado
salt and pepper

Garnishes:
tomato, sliced
cucumber, sliced

fresh boiled beetroot, cubed
chopped chives or parsley
stuffed olives

puffed rice cakes (available from
health food shops)

Cut the avocado in half, remove the stone and scoop the flesh out of the jacket. Mash the flesh and season to taste. Halve or quarter the rice cakes with a sharp knife and spread with the mashed avocado. Decorate with any of the suggested garnishes.

An alternative   Feta cheese can also be served sliced on rice cakes and decorated.   (see photograph, page 42)

Melon and grape savoury starter

Serves 2–3   See photograph, page 42

half a 450 g/1 lb honeydew melon,
   chilled
60 g/2 oz black grapes, chilled
1½ tsp apple juice

3 tsp sunflower oil
salt and pepper
chopped chives

Scrape the seeds out of the melon, and either scoop out balls with a special cutter, or cube the flesh. Halve the grapes, removing pips if necessary. Mix the apple juice, oil, seasoning and chives. Pour over the fruit, toss and serve immediately (otherwise the dark grapes may discolour the melon).

Avocado provençal

Serves 2

20 g/⅔ oz green pepper, chopped
20 g/⅔ oz cucumber, chopped
1 tsp concentrated tomato purée
3 tsp apple juice
½ small clove garlic, finely sliced or
   crushed through press

1 avocado
salt and pepper
⅛ cayenne pepper
1 tbsp chopped parsley to garnish

Place the green pepper and cucumber in a small bowl. Make a dressing of the tomato purée, apple juice, garlic and seasoning. Pour over and stir together well. Cover with plastic film and leave in the refrigerator for 30 minutes to allow the flavours to blend (but not so long that the salads lose their crunchiness).

Cut the avocado in two, remove stone, fill the hollows with mixture, and serve garnished with fresh parsley.

Sophisticated swiss roll   W̅ M̅

Serves 6 as a starter   See photograph, page 42

225 g/8 oz frozen chopped spinach   *4 medium-size eggs*
30 g/1 oz Tomor margarine   *2 ripe avocado pears*
salt and pepper   *1–2 tsp apple juice*
½ tsp grated nutmeg

Preheat oven to 180 °C/350 °F/gas 4.

Line a 30 cm/12 in swiss roll tin with greaseproof paper rubbed with a little Tomor.

Heat the spinach in a pan with the Tomor, salt and pepper to taste, and nutmeg.

Separate the eggs: beat the whites until they hold peaks and the yolks until creamy.

Beat the spinach mixture into the yolks, then fold in the whites. Pour into the prepared tin and spread evenly with a spatula.

Bake for 20 minutes or until the top is just firm.

Cool in the tin to room temperature then cool further in the refrigerator for 30–60 minutes. Cover with a damp cloth and leave at room temperature for a further 30 minutes. Invert tin on to a board so that the swiss roll comes out with the cloth underneath. Peel off the greaseproof paper.

Scoop out the avocado flesh and mash with salt and pepper and as much apple juice as required to give a consistency that will spread easily.

Spread it on the baked mixture and carefully roll it up by holding up the edges of the cloth.

Bortsch   ✶ W̅ M̅ E̅

Serves 3   See photograph, page 44

450 g/1 lb raw beetroot   *salt and pepper*
2 sticks celery, chopped   *chopped chives and goat's or sheep's*
900 ml/1½ pint meat stock (see   *yoghurt to garnish*
* page 79)*

Peel and coarsely grate the beetroot into a pan. Add the celery, stock and seasoning. Bring to the boil and simmer uncovered for 45 minutes. Strain and adjust seasoning. Serve in bowls, garnished with yoghurt and chives.

NB To avoid staining your hands wear rubber gloves when peeling and grating the beetroot.

Celeriac soup   ⊠ W M E
Serves 2

1 celeriac – about tennis-ball size –   *salt and pepper*
peeled and cubed   *parsley to garnish*
300 ml/½ pint milk substitute

Put celeriac in a pan with milk substitute and 150 ml/¼ pint water. Bring to the boil and simmer for 10–15 minutes, or until cooked. Liquidize and strain the mixture. Adjust seasoning – extra salt takes away any bitterness – and reheat.
Serve garnished with a sprig of parsley.

Chestnut soup   ⊠ W M E
Serves 4   See photograph, page 44

170 g/6 oz dried chestnuts, soaked for   *½ grated nutmeg*
24 hours (see below)   *salt and pepper*
2 onions, roughly chopped   *150–300 ml/¼–½ pint milk sub-*
2 carrots, diced   *stitute*
2 sticks celery, diced   *parsley to garnish*
⅛ tsp thyme

Put chestnuts in a bowl. Pour over 1.2 litres/2 pints boiling water and leave soaking for at least 24 hours. Put chestnuts and liquid in a saucepan and add onions, carrots and celery. Simmer for about 1½ hours or until chestnuts are soft; or cook for ½ hour in pressure cooker. Liquidize, return to saucepan, add herbs and salt and pepper to taste, and thin down with milk.
Reheat to serve, but do not boil. Garnish with parsley before serving.

Chicken and mushroom soup
Serves 2   ⊠ W M E

1 chicken carcase   *300 ml/½ pint vegetable stock (see*
salt and pepper   *page 79)*
100 g/3½ oz mushrooms, chopped   *60 ml/2 fl oz milk substitute*
30 g/1 oz red lentils

Boil the carcase in 300 ml (½ pint) water with seasonings for 1–1½ hours or 15–20 minutes in a pressure cooker at high pressure. Remove bones and skin from the stock.

Add the mushrooms, lentils and vegetable stock. Cook for a further 20 minutes or 5 minutes in a pressure cooker. Adjust seasoning. Stir in milk and serve immediately.

Gazpacho

Serves 3

½ medium cucumber, chopped
225 g/½ lb ripe tomatoes, skinned
  and chopped
60 g/2 oz green or red pepper,
  chopped

1 clove garlic, crushed
1 tbsp sunflower oil
1 tbsp concentrated tomato purée
salt and pepper
chives to garnish

Mix all the ingredients in a bowl with 200 ml/7 fl oz water and purée in an electric blender.

Transfer to serving dish and chill covered with plastic film for 1–2 hours.

If too thick, dilute with a little iced water or a couple of ice cubes. Serve garnished with chopped chives.

Leek soup

Serves 3–4

2 medium size leeks, chopped
4 small carrots, chopped
150 ml/¼ pint milk substitute

salt and pepper
2 tbsp chopped cooked chicken
  (optional)

Cook the vegetables in 300 ml/½ pint salted water for 10–15 minutes or until tender. Liquidize, and return to the pan, adding the milk substitute and adjusting the seasoning. Add the chicken if used. Bring to the boil, simmer and cook for 2 or 3 minutes. Serve.

Quick snack lunch soup

Serves 1

50 g/1½ oz carrot, chopped
50 g/1½ oz celery, chopped
20 g/⅔ oz red lentils

salt and pepper to taste
2 tsp tomato purée
parsley to garnish

Simmer all the ingredients together in 300 ml/½ pint water for 20 minutes or until soft. Liquidize. Reheat. Serve garnished with parsley.

Tomato and courgette soup

Serves 4 ★ W M E

225 g/8 oz courgettes, trimmed
225 g/8 oz ripe tomatoes, skinned
1050 ml/1¾ pint milk substitute
1 tbsp chopped parsley
sprig thyme
salt and pepper

Steam the courgettes until tender. Chop and mix with tomatoes, milk, parsley, thyme leaves, salt and pepper to taste. Purée in liquidizer. Put in a pan, bring to the boil, adjust seasoning and serve. (see photograph, page 44)

An alternative This can also be served as an iced summer soup: chill the mixture and, if you like, add ice cubes before serving.

SALADS AND VEGETABLES

Apple and bean salad ★ W M E

Serves 4

450 g/1 lb shelled broad beans, fresh or frozen, cooked and allowed to cool
1 Granny Smith apple, cored and chopped
2 tbsp olive oil
2 tbsp apple juice
1½ tsp chopped parsley
1½ tsp chopped chives
salt and freshly ground black pepper

Mix the beans and apple in a big bowl. Add the olive oil, apple juice, herbs and seasoning and stir well.

Cover and leave to marinade in the refrigerator for 2–3 hours, stirring occasionally, before serving.

This is a convenient and appetizing addition to a lunch box.

The devil's own drumsticks (*top*, see page 65), Apple and bean salad (*bottom*)

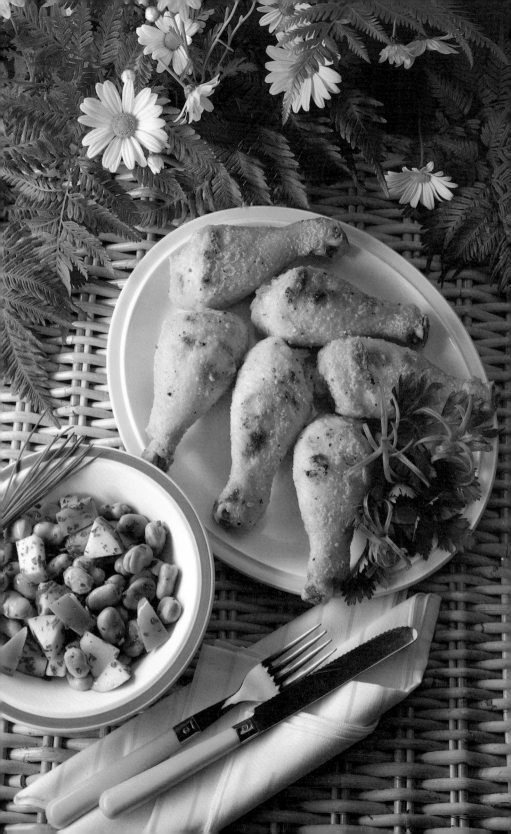

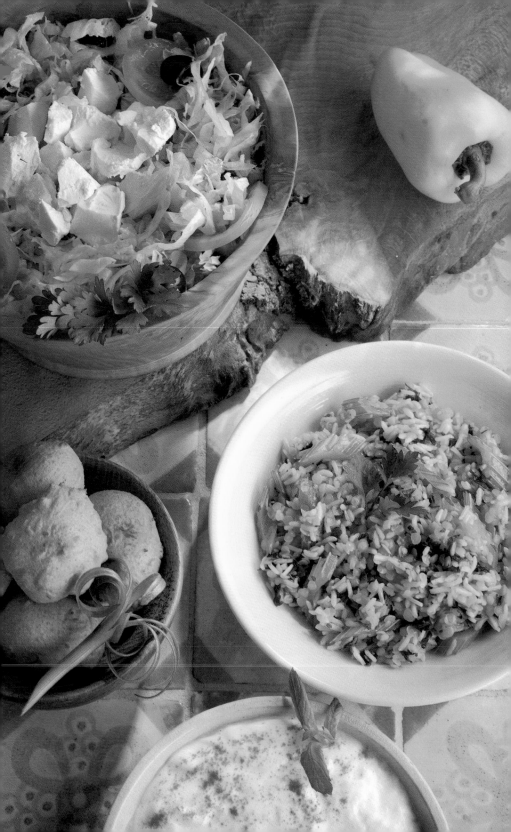

Chick pea salad

Serves 2–4

240 g/8 oz chick peas, soaked over-
night in water
30 ml/1 fl oz olive oil

2 cloves garlic, crushed
salt and pepper
1 tbsp chopped parsley to garnish

Drain the chick peas, put in a large saucepan, cover with water, bring to boil and simmer for 3–3½ hours, or cook in a pressure cooker for 15 minutes at high pressure.

Stir in the oil, garlic and seasoning. Serve hot or cold, garnished with parsley.

An alternative Skinned and sliced tomatoes can also be added to the salad.

Chicken Waldorf

Serves 2

150–200 g/5–7 oz cold cooked
  chicken, chopped
2 sticks celery, chopped
1 eating apple, cored and chopped

60 g/2 oz walnuts, chopped
salt and freshly ground black pepper
75 ml/2½ fl oz goat's yoghurt
watercress to garnish

Combine the chicken, celery, apple and nuts in a serving bowl. Season, add the yoghurt and toss. Garnish with watercress.

Feta salad

Serves 4

225 g/8 oz feta cheese
1 crisp lettuce
60 g/2 oz black olives
225 g/½ lb tomatoes

Dressing:
2 tbsp olive oil
2 cloves garlic, crushed
salt and pepper

The cheese can be crumbled into the salad or served separately.

Finely chop the lettuce and mix with olives and sliced tomatoes. Mix oil, garlic and seasoning and pour over salad. Toss and serve.

NB Add lemon juice to the dressing if allowed.

Feta salad (*top*), Brown rice and lentils (*centre right*, see page 61), Pakoras (*centre left*, see page 59), Raita (*bottom*, see page 86)

Curried rice salad

Serves 4–6

225 g/8 oz brown rice

¼ tsp cayenne pepper (optional)

Dressing:
2 tbsp sunflower oil
½ tbsp apple juice
curry powder (make sure it is wheat-
free) to taste (about 3 tsp)*

170 g/6 oz apple, chopped
60 g/2 oz walnuts, chopped
60 g/2 oz sultanas or raisins
120 g/4 oz red or green pepper,
chopped

Cook the rice (see page 25). Drain. In a bowl, stir the dressing ingredients together. Pour over the rice while still warm and mix well. Add the other salad ingredients when the rice is cool and toss lightly.

Alternatives   Add celery, cucumber, bananas.

Sweet salad   M E

Serves 2

60 g/2 oz kohl rabi or swede
100 g/3½ oz small cauliflower florets
1 handful sultanas

salt and freshly ground black pepper
2 tbsp sheep's yoghurt cheese
sliced mushrooms to garnish

Coarsely grate the kohl rabi and mix with the florets. Add the sultanas and seasoning.

In a separate bowl mix the cheese with 60 ml/2 fl oz water to produce a thin paste. Pour over the vegetable mixture and stir well. Chill for 1 hour. Stir again and garnish with the mushrooms, ready to serve.

This is a handy and filling snack to put in a lunch box.

Cabbage in the Chinese style W M E

Serves 4

1 tbsp sunflower oil
1 clove garlic, crushed
½ large white cabbage, shredded
1 tsp demerara sugar
salt and pepper

⅛ tsp paprika
100 g/3½ oz chopped almonds
15 g/½ oz root ginger, peeled and
finely chopped

Heat the oil in a saucepan and fry the garlic until golden. Add the cabbage, sugar, salt, pepper, paprika and 4 tbsp water. Simmer

---

*If you prefer, the curry powder can be cooked before adding: heat 2 tsp oil and fry 1 crushed clove garlic and 3 tsp curry powder very gently for 2 minutes. Turn this into the rice with all the other ingredients.

gently, removing lid to stir occasionally for 5–10 minutes, until the cabbage is nearly cooked. Add almonds and ginger and cook for another couple of minutes.
Serve hot.

Glazed carrots W M E

Serves 2

60 g/2 oz Tomor margarine
450 g/1 lb young carrots scraped and
  left whole
3 tsp sugar
30 g/1 oz brown rice miso dissolved in

300 ml/½ pint hot, not boiling
  water
freshly ground pepper
chopped parsley to garnish

Melt Tomor in a saucepan. Add carrots, sugar, salt and enough miso mixture to come half way up the carrots. Cook gently without a lid, stirring occasionally until soft. Remove carrots and keep hot.
  Boil liquid rapidly until reduced to a rich glaze. Roll the carrots in it until they are well coated. Season with pepper and garnish with parsley.

Chinese-style cauliflower and runner beans

Serves 2

225 g/8 oz runner beans (fresh or
  frozen), strings removed and sliced
¼ average size cauliflower (fresh or
  frozen), broken into florets
4 tbsp sunflower oil

12 blanched almonds
1 clove garlic, crushed
1 tsp sugar
1 tsp paprika
salt and pepper

Cook vegetables in salted water for 5 minutes and drain.
  Heat oil in a large frying pan and fry the almonds and garlic for 1 minute or until golden.
  Add beans and cauliflower, sugar, paprika and seasoning to taste. Fry, stirring over a low heat for 2–3 minutes.

Parsnip chips W M E

Serves 2

170–225 g/6–8 oz unprepared
  parsnips per person

sunflower oil as required
salt and pepper

Peel the parsnips and cut into rounds about 5 mm/¼ in thick. Cover the base of a heavy-based frying pan with oil. Heat the oil and when it is medium hot, slip in the parsnip slices and let them sizzle briefly. Turn down heat and let them cook through, then turn up heat and brown them (the whole process should take less than 5 minutes).

Drain on kitchen paper, season to taste and serve immediately.

Creamed spinach

Serves 2

675 g/1½ lb spinach   60 m/2 fl oz milk substitute
60 g/2 oz Tomor margarine   ½ tsp ground nutmeg

Wash and drain the spinach well. Cook in a large pan with the Tomor margarine. Cook for 10 minutes or until the spinach is soft and the fluid reduced. Add nutmeg and milk substitute, and continue cooking until the spinach is almost dry but still creamy.

Baked sweet potatoes

Serves 4–6

450 g/1 lb sweet potatoes, peeled   ⅛ tsp salt
  and diced   ¼ tsp ground ginger
150 ml/¼ pt milk substitute   ¼ tsp ground cinnamon
2 eggs   1 tbsp brown rice miso, mixed to a paste
60 ml/2 fl oz oil (sunflower, safflower,   with a little water
  soya)   4 tbsp honey

Preheat the oven to 180 °C/350 °F/gas 4.

Liquidize all the ingredients together briefly so that you have a coarse mixture. Put in a greased casserole dish and bake for 45 minutes.

This is a sweet vegetable which goes very well with pork or chicken dishes.

An alternative   Yams can be used instead of sweet potatoes.

VEGETARIAN DISHES

Pakoras ☒ Ⓦ Ⓜ Ⓔ

Serves 4   See photograph, page 54

Batter: Vegetables – use one or a com-
225 g/8 oz gram flour   bination of the following:
½ tsp commercial wheat-free baking   diced stalks and florets of cauliflower
  powder (see page 89)   diced aubergines
1 tsp salt   onion rings
½ tsp ground coriander
1 tsp garam masala   oil for frying (soya, sunflower,
½ tsp chilli powder   safflower)
½tsp ground cumin

Sieve all the dry ingredients into a bowl. Add sufficient water
(about 300 ml/½ pint) water to make a thick batter and beat well.
Add the vegetables to the batter mixture.
   Deep fry the pakoras: drop 1 tbsp of batter mixture at a time
into the medium hot oil (do not overcrowd the pan) and cook
until golden brown.
   Drain and serve immediately with salad and raita (see page
86).

NB For those who like spicy food, the quantity of spices can be
increased in the batter mixture.

Légumes au gratin ☒ Ⓦ Ⓜ Ⓔ

Serves 4

1 cauliflower broken into florets (fresh   salt
  or 450 g/1 lb frozen)   120 g/4 oz bean sprouts
3 large carrots, peeled and slit in   200 g/7 oz feta cheese, grated
  rounds   sliced tomato and chopped parsley to
120 g/4 oz brussels sprouts (fresh or   garnish
  frozen)

Cook all the vegetables except the bean sprouts in boiling salted
water until just firm to bite. Drain and put into a shallow fireproof
dish with the bean sprouts. Sprinkle with grated cheese.
   Place under the grill until the cheese is browned.
   Serve garnished with tomato and parsley.

Mediterranean vegetables

Serves 2

340 g/12 oz courgettes, finely sliced
200 g/7 oz small aubergines, finely
   sliced
salt and pepper
30–60 g/1–2 oz Tomor margarine

340 g/12 oz tomatoes, skinned and
   sliced
dried thyme and basil
60 g/2 oz feta cheese
30 ml/1 oz olive oil

Preheat oven to 200 °C/400 °F/gas 6.

Season courgettes and aubergines and sauté separately in the Tomor. Season tomatoes.

Grease a small casserole with Tomor and layer the vegetables – at least 2 layers of each – ending with a layer of courgettes. Sprinkle with a pinch of thyme and basil. Crumble the feta cheese on top and pour the olive oil over the mixture.

Bake for 15–20 minutes.

Stuffed tomatoes

Serves 2–4

675 g/1½ lb tomatoes – 4 large
   tomatoes or 2 large beefsteak
salt and pepper
120 g/4 oz brown rice
1 stick celery, grated
1 medium green pepper, cored and
   finely chopped

2 cloves garlic, crushed
15 g/½ oz Tomor margarine
handful of parsley, chopped
1 tbsp chopped mint
1 tbsp currants, chopped
30 ml/1 fl oz olive oil

Cut the tops off the tomatoes and set them aside. Scoop out the pulp and set that aside (take care not to remove too much flesh or the tomatoes will split when cooked). Sprinkle the tomato shells lightly with salt, invert them and let them drain.

Preheat oven to 180 °C/350 °F/gas 4.

Part cook rice in boiling water until it begins to soften. Drain.

Fry the celery, pepper, and garlic gently in Tomor margarine until almost done. Chop the tomato pulp and add it with herbs, seasonings and currants. Simmer for 3 minutes and take off heat. Add rice to this mixture, strain off most of the excess juice and reserve.

Stuff the tomatoes with the rice and vegetable mixture and replace the reserved tops. Arrange in shallow baking dish. Add the olive oil to the reserved juice to make a gravy and pour it round the stuffed tomatoes.

Cook for 40 minutes in the oven, basting occasionally to prevent the outsides from drying out.

Serve hot or cold as a snack meal or accompaniment to another dish.

Brown rice and lentils   ✶ W M E

Serves 2–4   See photograph, page 54

225 g/8 oz brown rice
170 g/6 oz red lentils
2 sticks celery, chopped
1 clove garlic, crushed
1 handful parsley, chopped

1 tbsp oil (sunflower, safflower, soya)
½ tsp sea salt
½ tsp ground cumin
2 tbsp brown rice miso, mixed to a paste
  with a little water

Cook rice (see page 25). Drain.
   Wash lentils and cook for 15 minutes in 900 ml/1½ pints water.
Sauté celery, garlic and parsley in oil. Add rice and vegetables to
the lentils and simmer until thick. Add salt, cumin and miso to
taste.
   Serve hot with a salad.

Alternatives   Any allowed vegetables can be added.
   Leftovers can be shaped into rounds and fried in oil to make
burgers.

Buckwheat croquettes   ✶ W M E

Serves 2

170 g/6 oz buckwheat
2 sticks celery, grated
30 g/1 oz soya flour

salt and pepper
herbs as desired, eg, parsley, sage
2 tbsp oil

Cook buckwheat (see page 25). Drain and cool. Add celery, soya
flour, seasonings and herbs, and stir until evenly mixed. Shape
into 1 cm/½ in-thick rounds. Fry in oil, on both sides, until
cooked.
   Serve with apple sauce or tomato sauce (see page 85), or tahini
gravy (see page 80).

Red bean lasagne   W M

Serves 4–6

225 g/8 oz kidney beans, soaked in
  water overnight
1 large onion, chopped
1 tbsp oil
450 g/1 lb tomatoes, skinned and
  chopped
2 sticks celery, grated

4 whole cloves
1 tbsp chopped fresh majoram or
  1 tsp dried
2 cloves garlic, crushed
salt and pepper
120 g/4 oz feta cheese, crumbled
buckwheat pasta (see page 63)

Drain the beans. Put in a large pan with plenty of fresh water and
boil for 1–1½ hours or cook in a pressure cooker for 15 minutes at
high pressure. Drain.

Fry the onion in the oil until soft. Add all the other ingredients, except the beans and cheese, simmer in a covered pan for 10 minutes. Mix in the beans.

Preheat oven to 180 °C/350 °F/gas 4.

Make the pasta using half the quantities given on page 63, that is, a total of 120 g/4 oz flour. Roll out and cut into oblong sheets.

Cook the pasta in boiling water for 2–3 minutes. Remove each sheet individually from the pan and drain (if drained together in a colander they will stick together). Grease a shallow dish and arrange in it layers of bean mixture, cheese and pasta, ending with beans and cheese. Bake for 30 minutes.

Alternatives   1. For a moister dish, make a sauce using milk substitute thickened with rice flour and layer this with the bean mixture and cheese.

2. Make a filling of cooked spinach with feta cheese, and top with a white sauce and grated cheese.

Stuffed aubergines   [W] [M] [E]

Serves 2

2 *large aubergines*	1 *small onion, chopped*
sesame seeds	30 *g/1 oz millet flakes*
olive oil	½ *tsp dried basil*
450 *g/1 lb tomatoes, skinned and*	*salt and pepper*
chopped	60 *g/2 oz feta cheese*
3 *cloves garlic, crushed*	

Preheat oven to 200 °C/400 °F/gas 6.

Cut aubergines lengthways, lay in an ovenproof dish, and sprinkle with sesame seeds and a little oil. Bake for about 20 minutes, or until soft. Cool a little and scoop out middle; chop this pulp.

Simmer tomatoes, garlic, onion, millet, herbs and seasoning for 10 minutes. Mix with aubergine pulp.

Fill the shells with this mixture and top with crumbled feta cheese. Bake for 30 minutes until heated through and the cheese has melted.

Serve with salad.

Ratatouille   [✱] [W] [M] [E]

Serves 4

3 *cloves garlic, crushed*	400 *g/14 oz tomatoes, skinned*
1 *large or 2 small aubergines, sliced*	1 *tsp honey*
1 *large green pepper, sliced*	*salt and freshly ground black pepper*
60 *g/2 oz cucumber, sliced*	5 *tbsp olive oil*
225 *g/8 oz courgettes, sliced*	

Season the vegetables generously with black pepper and lightly with salt. Add the honey and simmer them gently in the oil in a pan with a closely fitting lid for approximately 1 hour, stirring occasionally.

Buckwheat pasta   W M

Serves 4

225 g/8 oz buckwheat flour   *1 small egg*
22 g/¾ oz Tomor margarine   *salt*

Sift the flour into a bowl and make a well in the centre. Put in the Tomor, egg and a pinch of salt. Mix thoroughly, adding a little water to make a thick dough. Knead well until the dough is smooth. If the mixture is too sticky, add more flour.
    Roll out the dough on a lightly floured surface, using buckwheat or rice flour, until the pasta is very thin. Cut into required shapes.
    Put the pasta into a large pan containing plenty of salted boiling water. A little oil can be added to the water to prevent the pasta from sticking together. Boil uncovered for 3–5 minutes, until just tender but firm to bite. Do not overcook.
    Drain in a colander and serve immediately.
    Good served with a sauce, such as meat sauce, cheese or tomato, or lasagne, above.

An alternative   If you find the taste of buckwheat too strong, use half rice flour and half buckwheat.

SNACKS

Baked beans   ✱ W M E

Serves 2–4

225 g/8 oz haricot beans, soaked *300 ml/½ pint basic tomato sauce (see*
    overnight in cold water   *page 85)*
                      salt and pepper

Drain the beans and put in a large pan with plenty of water. Boil for 1–1½ hours or cook in pressure cooker for 6 minutes at high pressure. Drain. Mix with the tomato sauce, adjust seasoning and heat through.

Can be served hot or cold.

NB Chilli powder can be added to the sauce if liked.

Butter bean brunch

Serves 2

100 g/3½ oz butter beans, soaked in cold water overnight
2 tbsp sunflower oil
225 g/½ lb tomatoes, coarsely chopped

100 g/3½ oz green pepper, seeded and chopped
30 g/1 oz brown rice miso, mixed to a paste with a little water
60 g/2 oz mushrooms, chopped
salt and pepper

Drain the beans and put in a large pan with plenty of water. Boil for 1–1½ hours or cook in a pressure cooker for 10 minutes at high pressure. Drain.

Heat the oil in a pan and fry the tomatoes and peppers gently for 10 minutes. Add the beans, miso mixture, mushrooms and seasoning and simmer for another 10 minutes.

Italian tomatoes

Sufficient to cover 4 slices bread

340 g/¾ lb tomatoes
3 cloves garlic, crushed

½ tbsp olive oil
chopped fresh basil to garnish

Pour boiling water over the tomatoes, then drain after 1 minute. Plunge into cold water, drain and peel. Chop the tomatoes, add the garlic and oil, and cook on low heat for 10 minutes.

Serve on wheat-free toast sprinkled with chopped basil.

Pizza

Serves 2

280 g/10 oz rice flour
½ tsp salt
15 g/½ oz fresh yeast or 7 g/¼ oz dried yeast
1 egg
olive oil

Filling:
tomato sauce (see page 85), anchovies, black olives, peppers, feta cheese, dried oregano

Put the flour and salt in a mixing bowl. Crumble in the yeast. Beat the egg and add it to the flour with enough lukewarm water to make a stiff dough. Press the dough into 2 round greased tins, 23 cm/9 in in diameter. Brush the tops with olive oil.

Layer the filling generously over the pizza base and sprinkle with oregano.

Preheat oven to 230 °C/450 °F/gas 8.

Allow pizzas to rise. Bake for 10 minutes, then turn oven down to 200 °C/400 °F/gas 6, and cook for a further 25 minutes.

Serve with a salad.

The devil's own drumsticks

As many chicken drumsticks as re-   *cayenne pepper to taste*
quired (thaw thoroughly if frozen)   *salt and pepper*
gram flour for coating

Coat the drumsticks in gram flour seasoned with salt, pepper and cayenne. Grill for 20–30 minutes, turning frequently.

Serve hot or cold.

These are especially good to take on picnics or to work for lunch. (see photograph, page 53)

FISH

Quick cod in mushroom sauce

Serves 2

2 frozen cod steaks
30 g/1 oz Tomor margarine

Sauce:
15 g/½ oz Tomor margarine
15 g/½ oz soya flour

120 ml/4 fl oz milk substitute
100 g/3½ oz button mushrooms, sliced
salt and pepper
parsley to garnish

Dot the frozen cod with Tomor and grill for about 6 minutes on each side.

To make sauce, melt the Tomor and make a roux by adding the flour, then gradually stir in the milk. Add the mushrooms and season to taste. Simmer and stir for a couple of minutes.

Put the cod steaks on a warmed serving dish and pour the sauce over them. Garnish with fresh parsley if available.

Flaked fish with vegetable rice   ✱ W M E

Serves 2

170 g/6 oz brown rice
225 g/8 oz white fish
170 g/6 oz cooked vegetables (eg, peas,
* diced carrots, chopped celery)*

1 handful parsley, chopped
30 g/1 oz Tomor margarine
cayenne pepper
sea salt

Cook the rice (see page 25) and drain.
Poach the fish in water for 10 minutes. Remove skin and bones and flake it. Combine the fish, rice, vegetables and parsley and heat in the Tomor. Add seasoning to taste.
Serve hot.

Crispy coated fish   ✱ W M E

Serves 2

12 tbsp millet
2 haddock fillets, about 280 g/10 oz

milk substitute
salt and pepper

Lightly grind the millet in a coffee grinder until it resembles breadcrumbs. Moisten the fillets with milk substitute, then roll them in the millet. Fry in oil.

Alternatives   Any other fish fillet, such as cod or plaice can be used.

Stuffed mackerel   ✱ W M E

Serves 2

2 medium size apples – about 150 g/
* 5 oz, peeled, cored and sliced*
85 g/3 oz celery, washed and chopped
1–2 tsp sunflower oil
salt and pepper

30 g/1 oz lightly ground millet
2 mackerel, boned
150 ml/¼ pint apple juice
1 level tsp arrowroot
1 level tsp sugar

Preheat oven to 180 °C/350 °F/gas 4.
Fry apples and celery in oil until the apples are soft. Season and stir in the millet.
Spread this stuffing inside each fish and place in an ovenproof dish with a little of the apple juice.
Cook in oven for 25–30 minutes. When almost ready, mix the arrowroot and sugar with a little of the apple juice. Heat the rest of the apple juice and stir into the paste, then return it all to the heat, until it thickens and clears.
Pour a little of the glaze over the fish; serve the rest separately as a sauce.

Mackerel with gooseberry   ⊠ W M E

Serves 2

2 mackerel fillets	*100 g/3½ oz gooseberries – fresh,*
4 tbsp lightly ground millet	*frozen or Hazlewoods' bottled*
salt and pepper	*1 tsp sugar*
knob of Tomor margarine	*⅛ tsp grated nutmeg*

Wash and dry mackerel fillets. Season ground millet and sprinkle over mackerel. Dot with the Tomor and cook under a preheated grill 15–20 minutes.

Stew the gooseberries, with 1 tbsp water, sugar and nutmeg. Rub through a sieve to remove the seeds.

Place mackerel on a warmed serving dish and pour over the gooseberry sauce. Serve immediately.

This dish is good served with courgettes and fresh small carrots.

Simple trout   ⊠ W M E

Serves 1   See photograph, page 71

15 g/½ oz Tomor margarine	*salt and pepper*
1–2 tbsp chopped parsley	*1 trout, gutted and cleaned*

Mix the Tomor, parsley and seasoning into a soft ball. Place most of the mixture inside the fish and dot the remainder on the outside. Grill under a moderate heat, 5–10 minutes on each side.

Serve with fresh green vegetables.

Baked salmon   ⊠ W M E

Serves 6

900 g/2 lb piece of salmon	*salt and pepper*
Tomor margarine	*chopped parsley*

Preheat oven to 150 °C /300 °F /gas 2.

Wipe the fish, removing the fins and any blood by the backbone. Grease a large piece of cooking foil with Tomor. Place the fish in the centre, season it lightly with salt and pepper and scatter the parsley over it. Wrap it loosely in the foil, and place on a baking sheet. Bake for 1¼–1¾ hours, depending on the thickness of the fish, but be careful not to overcook.

Serve hot. If you want to serve it cold, remove the skin while the fish is still warm.

Serve with a salad.

MEAT

Chilli con carne

Serves 2

150 g/5 oz dried red kidney beans,
  soaked overnight in cold water
225 g/8 oz minced beef
½ average size green pepper,
  coarsely chopped

4 tomatoes
1 green chilli, seeded and chopped
30 ml/1 fl oz tomato purée
salt and pepper

Heat a heavy bottomed casserole or pan and brown the meat. Drain and add the beans, green pepper, tomatoes and chilli. Stir in the tomato purée and enough water to cover, bring to the boil, boil for 10 minutes, then turn down heat and and simmer for 1½ hours or until the beans are cooked.

Alternatively, cook the beans separately in advance (1–1½ hours in boiling water, or 10 minutes in a pressure cooker at high pressure), then add to the cooked chilli and reheat.

Risotto with beef

Serves 2

60 g/2 oz Tomor margarine
2 sticks celery, cleaned and chopped
225 g/8 oz minced beef
225 g/8 oz brown rice, washed
⅛ tsp nutmeg

sea salt and pepper
1 tsp dried basil
120 g/4 oz tomatoes, chopped
2 tbsp brown rice miso mixed to a thick
  paste with a little water

Heat the Tomor in a saucepan. Sauté the celery and minced beef. When the beef has browned, add the rice and heat gently for about 10 minutes. Stir occasionally.

Sprinkle in the nutmeg, salt and pepper and basil. Cover with water and add the tomatoes. Cook gently for 45 minutes, adding more water if necessary to prevent the mixture drying out. When the rice is cooked and the water absorbed, stir in the miso.

Serve hot with salad.

Liver with thyme and garlic

Serves 4

1–4 tbsp sunflower oil (as needed)
1 clove garlic, thinly sliced
450 g/1 lb lamb's liver, thinly sliced

1½ tsp dried thyme
salt and pepper
1 tbsp apple juice

Heat the oil and fry the garlic in it for a couple of minutes. Add the liver and brown quickly on both sides. Add the thyme, salt, pepper and apple juice and mix well. Cook for another minute, and serve immediately.

Bombay burgers   ⊠ Ⓦ Ⓜ Ⓔ

Serves 2

225 g/½ lb minced beef
¼ medium green pepper, finely
*   chopped*
1 clove garlic, crushed
1½ tsp concentrated tomato purée
3 tsp gram flour

⅛ tsp each of: ground cumin, chilli
*   powder, coriander, cinnamon, ginger,*
*   nutmeg and cloves*
salt and pepper
30 ml/1 fl oz apple juice

Put the meat, green pepper, garlic, tomato purée, 1½ tsp flour, spices, salt and pepper in a bowl and mix well, adding enough apple juice to give the mixture a firm consistency. Shape into burgers and dust with the remaining gram flour.

Cook under preheated grill for 10–15 minutes, turning occasionally until browned.

Serve with rice and a salad.

Four-meat pâté   ⊠ Ⓦ Ⓜ Ⓔ

12 generous portions

675 g/1½ lb lamb's liver
225 g/½ lb chicken liver
225 g/½ lb lean veal
450 g/1 lb belly pork
100 g/3½ oz green pepper
100 g/3½ oz mushrooms

2 cloves garlic
2 level tsp salt
2 level tsp fresh ground black pepper
2 level tsp dried basil
1–2 tomatoes, sliced

Preheat the oven to 180 °C/350 °F/gas 4.

Mince all the meats, the green pepper, mushrooms and garlic. Mix well together, adding the salt, pepper and basil. Spoon the mixture into an ovenproof dish or dishes and top with slices of tomato. Cover with foil and place in a larger pan containing sufficient hot water to come half way up the side of the dish. Bake for 2½–3 hours. When cool, cover with fresh foil, weight down and leave in a cool place.

Served with buckwheat pancakes, savoury rice cakes and salad, or savoury buckwheat biscuits, this pâté is particularly useful for snacks and packed lunches.

Rosemary and garlic lamb

Serves 2

30 g/1 oz green pepper, chopped
1 large clove garlic, crushed
2 tbsp sunflower oil
170–200 g/6–7 oz cold cooked lamb,
  coarsely chopped
3 tsp millet flour

30 g/1 oz brown rice miso mixed to a
  thick paste with a little water
¼ tsp dried rosemary
salt and pepper
parsley to garnish

Fry the green pepper and garlic in the oil until soft. Add the meat, and fry a further 5 minutes. Stir in the flour, the miso and the rosemary and season to taste.

Simmer for 10–15 minutes then serve on brown rice, garnished with parsley.

Balkan chops

Serves 2

4 tbsp apple juice
1 tbsp sunflower oil
salt and pepper
⅛ tsp dried thyme
2 lamb chops

½ clove garlic, finely sliced
75 g/2½ oz plain goat's or ewe's
  yoghurt
1 tsp paprika

Preheat oven to 190 °C/375 °F/gas 5.

Mix together the apple juice, oil, seasoning and thyme. Marinade the chops in this mixture for 2–3 hours. Drain the chops and place in a shallow ovenproof dish with the sliced garlic. Cover with foil and bake for 45–60 minutes or until cooked through.

Pour any gravy from around the chops into a bowl, skim off fat and keep hot.

Mix the yoghurt and paprika and spoon over the chops. Return to the oven for 15 minutes, this time uncovered.

Serve garnished with a little paprika and hand the gravy separately.

Meaty marrow

Serves 4

225 g/8 oz minced beef
1 small aubergine, sliced
⅓ medium green pepper, chopped
4 tomatoes, chopped
120 g/¼ lb large button mushrooms,
  sliced

oregano and basil
salt and pepper
2 tsp concentrated tomato purée
half a large marrow
15 g/½ oz brown rice miso dissolved in
  150 ml/¼ pint hot water

Simple trout (*top*, see page 67), Balkan chops (*bottom*)

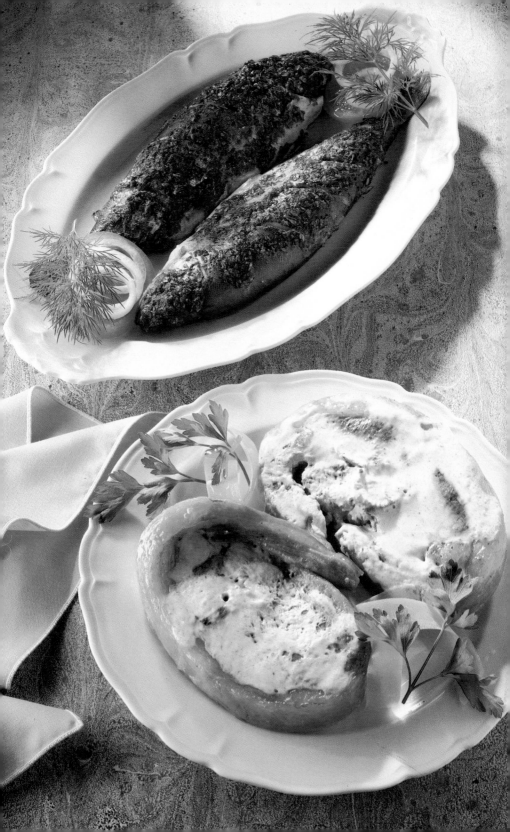

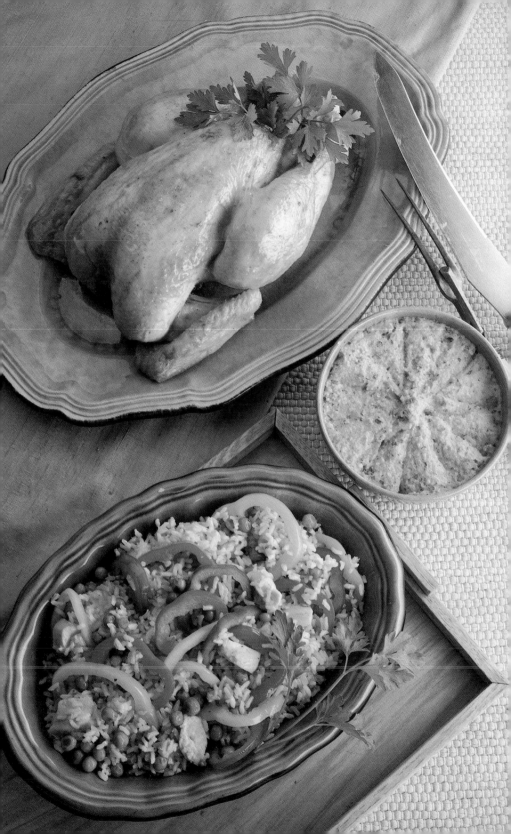

Heat the frying pan and fry the minced beef until browned. Move the meat to the side of the pan and fry the aubergine, green pepper, tomatoes and mushrooms in the resultant fat. Add the herbs and seasoning, and stir in the tomato purée.

Cut the marrow into thick slices. Peel, cut out the middle pith, and arrange on the base of a large casserole. Spoon the meat mixture into the middle of the marrow rings and pour over the miso. Cover well and simmer 45 minutes or until the marrow is tender.

Rabbit casserole

Serves 2

340–450 g/12–16 oz rabbit
2–4 carrots, peeled and cubed
4 prunes
4 or 6 large mushrooms, peeled and sliced
250 g/9 oz kohl rabi, swede or turnip,
*   peeled and cubed*
30 g/1 oz brown rice miso mixed to a
*   thick paste in a little water*
¼ tsp mixed herbs
salt and pepper
2–3 tsp millet flour

Preheat oven to 180 °C/350 °F/gas 4.

Place all the ingredients in a suitably sized casserole with 150 ml/¼ pint water and cook for 1¼–1½ hours.

Thicken the gravy by mixing the millet flour to a paste with a little water and stirring it in. Cook for a further ¼ hour.

Kidney supper

Serves 2

4 large or 6 small kidneys
½ medium green pepper, chopped
2 small cloves garlic, crushed
2 tbsp sunflower oil
4 medium carrots, peeled and sliced
4 tomatoes, quartered
30 g/1 oz brown rice miso mixed to a
*   thick paste with a little water*
salt and pepper
1½ tsp gram flour (optional)

Skin the kidneys, cut lengthways and remove the cores.

Fry the green pepper and garlic in the oil and then add the carrots and halved kidneys. When these are browned, add the tomatoes, miso, 300 ml/½ pint water and salt and pepper to taste. Simmer gently for 15 minutes or until cooked. If necessary thicken the sauce by mixing the gram flour into a paste with a little cold water, then tipping the hot sauce on to it. Stir well and return to the pan to cook for another 2 minutes.

Serve in a ring of rice.

Roast chicken with sweet potato stuffing (*top and centre*, see page 74), Amazing technicolour risotto (*bottom*, see page 75)

POULTRY AND GAME

Roast chicken with sweet potato stuffing

Serves 4   See photograph, page 72   ✱ W M E

Stuffing:

170 g/6 oz cooked sweet potato
30 g/1 oz lightly ground millet
sprig parsley, chopped
¼ tsp dried sage
salt and pepper
milk substitute

1 roasting chicken weighing about
  2 kg/4.4 lb
salt and pepper
vegetable oil (soya, sunflower,
  safflower)

Mash the sweet potato and stir in the millet, herbs, salt and pepper with enough milk substitute to give a firm consistency. Press into an oiled baking dish. Cover with foil.

Preheat oven to 200 °C/400 °F/gas 6.

Remove the giblets from the chicken and wipe inside and out. Season the inside of the bird lightly and spread the breast with a little vegetable oil. Place in a roasting tin and seal in the hot oven for 10 minutes. Then reduce the heat to 180 °C/350 °F/gas 4 and cover the chicken with foil.

Cook for a further 45–50 minutes, basting the chicken occasionally. Place the baking dish with the stuffing in the oven 30 minutes from the end of the cooking time.

Culpepper's chicken   ✱ W M E

Serves 2

1½ tbsp finely chopped parsley
2 large spikes chives, finely chopped
15 g/½ oz Tomor margarine

2 chicken joints
salt and pepper

Mash together the herbs and Tomor. Making only one entry point, lift the skin away from the flesh taking care not to break the skin. Gently pack half the herb mixture under the skin of each joint. Lightly season the other side of the joint and grill that first, then turn to grill the stuffed side (about 10 minutes on each side, or until done).

Amazing technicolour risotto

Serves 2　　See photograph, page 72

150 g/5 oz brown rice
15 ml/½ fl oz sunflower oil
1 clove garlic, crushed
100 g/3½ oz cooked chicken, chopped
60 g/2 oz each of green, red and yellow

peppers, sliced
30 g/1 oz mushrooms, sliced
3 tomatoes, chopped
100 g/3½ oz frozen peas
salt and pepper

Cook the rice (see page 25).

While the rice is cooking, heat the oil in a pan and fry the garlic, chicken, peppers and mushrooms. When the vegetables are soft, add the tomatoes, peas, and a little water and salt and pepper to taste. Cook over a gentle heat, stirring frequently. Add the rice when ready and mix well.

Serve with salad.

Caribbean chicken

Serves 2

2 chicken portions
salt and pepper
1 clove garlic, crushed
⅛ tsp dried rosemary and ground ginger

180 ml/6 oz unsweetened pineapple juice
1½ tsp millet flour to thicken sauce
chopped parsley to garnish

Preheat oven to 180 °C/350 °F/gas 4.

Put the chicken in a casserole dish, sprinkle with seasonings, garlic and herbs and pour over the pineapple juice.

Bake for approximately ¾ hour in the covered casserole.

Lift the chicken joints out and put under a hot grill to brown the skin. Meanwhile, mix the millet flour to a paste with a little water, add to the sauce and simmer for 1 minute. Pour the sauce over the chicken and garnish with parsley.

Serve with fresh green vegetables or a salad.

Chick pea chicken supper

Serves 2

100 g/3½ oz dry weight chick peas,
soaked overnight in water
30 g/1 oz brown rice miso dissolved in
300 ml/½ pint hot water
300 ml/½ pint apple juice
2 cloves garlic, crushed
¼ tsp dried rosemary

2 bay leaves
⅛ tsp cumin
225 g/½ lb pork leg steak, cubed
2 chicken drumsticks
salt and pepper
2 tbsp millet flour mixed to a paste
in water

Drain the chick peas and cook in plenty of boiling water for 1 hour (10 minutes in a pressure cooker at high pressure). They will not be completely cooked. Drain.

Mix all the ingredients together except for the millet flour and cook for 1¼–1½ hours, or 15 minutes in a pressure cooker. Thicken the gravy with the millet flour paste. Simmer uncovered for 5 minutes. Remove bay leaves and serve.

This dish is good served with spinach.

Spicy turkey

Serves 2

60 g/2 oz green pepper, coarsely chopped
45 g/1½ oz mushrooms, chopped
3 tbsp sunflower oil
2 turkey fillets
30 g/1 oz millet flour
⅛ tsp ground ginger

⅛ tsp ground nutmeg
15 g/½ oz brown rice miso dissolved in 150 ml/¼ pint warm water
60 ml/2 fl oz milk substitute
salt and pepper
toasted flaked almonds to garnish

Fry the green pepper and mushroom in the oil until soft. Move to one side of the pan and briskly fry the turkey until sealed.

Lift the turkey out and keep hot. Stir the millet, ginger and nutmeg into the oil, green pepper and mushroom mixture and cook for 1 minute. Gradually stir in the miso mixture and milk. Return the turkey and adjust the seasoning. Cover and simmer for 20–30 minutes or until the turkey is cooked through.

Serve garnished with the almonds.

Indian spiced chicken and tomatoes

Serves 2

2 tbsp sunflower oil
4 cloves garlic, crushed (or less according to taste)
280 g/10 oz boned raw chicken, cubed
1 tsp ground coriander
1 tsp cumin
½ tsp turmeric

¼ tsp cayenne pepper
225 g/8 oz tomatoes, skinned and coarsely chopped
90 ml/3 fl oz chicken stock (see page 79)
1 tsp garam masala
salt

Heat oil in frying pan and lightly brown the garlic. Add the chicken, coriander, cumin, turmeric and cayenne pepper and fry, stirring, for 1 minute. Add the tomatoes and squash to a pulp. Add chicken stock and simmer for 5 minutes or until the chicken is cooked through. Stir in the garam masala and salt to taste.

Serve with rice or gram flour flatbread (see page 91) and raita (see page 86).

Alternatives Any other meat can be substituted for chicken in the recipe.

Oriental chicken ⊠ Ⓦ Ⓜ Ⓔ

Serves 2

150 g/5 oz brown rice
1 tsp concentrated tomato purée
2 cloves garlic, crushed
2 portions chicken, boned and cubed
1 green chilli, seeded and finely chopped
60 g/2 oz okra, chopped

15–30 ml/½–1 oz sunflower oil
30 g/1 oz sultanas
3 tomatoes, chopped
¼ tsp ground ginger
salt and pepper
cucumber rings to garnish

Cook the rice (see page 25). When ready, stir in the tomato purée.

Fry the garlic, chicken, chilli and okra in the oil. When the chicken and okra are almost cooked, add 150 ml/¼ pint water, sultanas, tomatoes, ginger, salt and pepper and simmer until cooked through.

Serve the chicken in a ring of rice and garnish with cucumber rings.

Mango chutney is a good accompaniment. (Sharwood's is preservative and colouring-free).

Chicken liver with mushrooms ⊠ Ⓦ Ⓜ Ⓔ

Serves 4

340 g/12 oz chicken liver
1 tbsp sunflower oil
60 g/2 oz green pepper, chopped
15 g/½ oz green chilli, seeded and chopped
2 cloves garlic, crushed
1 tbsp gram flour
6–8 tomatoes, quartered

1 tbsp concentrated tomato purée dissolved in 100 ml/3½ fl oz water
1 tsp dried mixed herbs
salt and pepper
130 g/4½ oz button mushrooms, sliced
150 ml/5 fl oz apple juice

Remove any discoloured patches and fibres from the livers and chop them roughly.

Heat the oil in a pan, add the green pepper, chilli and garlic and cook until soft. Dust the chicken livers in seasoned gram flour. Move the green peppers and chilli to one side of the pan, and fry the livers quickly until lightly browned.

Add the tomatoes, tomato purée solution, herbs, salt and pepper. Bring to the boil and simmer uncovered for 20 minutes.

Add the mushrooms and apple juice and cook for a further 5–10 minutes.

This dish is good served on buckwheat pancakes (see page 45).

Turkey with apple and cherries

Serves 2   See photograph, page 81

2 turkey breasts
15 ml/½ fl oz sunflower oil
1 clove garlic, crushed
⅓ medium size green pepper, chopped
3 tsp gram flour
30 g/1 oz brown rice miso dissolved in
   300 ml/½ pint hot water

2 tbsp apple juice
2 tsp redcurrant jelly
1 medium size cooking apple, peeled
   and chopped
100 g/3½ oz cherries, washed and
   stoned
salt and pepper

Grill the turkey portions.

Heat the oil in a large frying pan and fry the garlic and green pepper for 1 minute. Turn down the heat and stir in the gram flour and cook for another minute. Stir the miso mixture gradually into the flour and green pepper paste. Stir in the apple juice and redcurrant jelly. Add the apple and cherries. Season with salt and pepper.

Transfer the turkey and its juices from the grill pan to the frying pan. Cover and simmer gently for a further 5–10 minutes.

Scarecrow's favourite

Serves 2

2 wood pigeons, plucked and drawn
(frozen birds are usually available)
30 g/1 oz Tomor margarine
60 g/2 oz chopped mushrooms
2 small bay leaves

1½ tbsp redcurrant jelly
6 peppercorns
salt and pepper
2 tbsp soya flour
watercress to garnish

Wash and dry the pigeons. Fry in Tomor until browned. Add mushrooms, bay leaves, redcurrant jelly, peppercorns, salt and pepper and about 600 ml/1 pint water. Cover and simmer for 1–1½ hours or until birds are cooked.

Remove the pigeons from the pan. Mix the soya flour to a paste with a little cold water and stir into the gravy. Simmer for a further 5 minutes.

Garnish the pigeons with watercress, and serve with the thickened gravy and extra redcurrant jelly.

STOCKS, BATTERS, SAUCES AND SALAD DRESSINGS

Stocks ☒ Ⓦ Ⓜ Ⓔ

Vegetable stock An economical substitute for stock is the water in which any allowed vegetables have been cooked.

Use vegetable leftovers and discards such as the outer leaves of cabbage or spinach. Wash and store in a refrigerator in a plastic bag. When ready to make stock, chop the vegetables, just cover with lightly salted water and boil slowly for fifteen minutes to extract flavours, vitamins and minerals. Strain off the liquid and cool.

Meat or chicken stock Use the raw bones of any suitable meat or poultry. Cover the bones with lightly salted cold water, bring to the boil and simmer for 3 hours, or cook in a pressure cooker for 30 minutes. Strain off the liquid and allow to cool, then lift off fat.

Store any unused stock in the refrigerator, or freeze it.

Gravies ☒ Ⓦ Ⓜ Ⓔ

Vegetable purées can be used in place of conventional gravy mixes such as Bisto, stock cubes or instant gravies. For convenience the purées can be made in bulk and frozen in smaller quantities for later use.

Examples
1. Red cabbage and mushrooms with sea salt and black pepper cooked with a blob of Tomor margarine and a little water until soft, then put through a blender, makes a rich replacement for gravy.
2. Skinned tomatoes, leeks, basil and sugar cooked together until soft, then put through a blender, makes a sweet sauce, ideal for lamb and minced beef dishes.
3. Carrots, celery and leeks with parsley cooked until soft, then put through a blender, makes a good accompaniment to chicken, turkey or egg dishes.

To colour gravies, sauces and soups use gravy browning made from caramelized sugar (see overleaf).

Gravy browning

Makes about 150 ml/¼ pint

120 g/4 oz sugar   *approximately 150 ml/5 fl oz water*

Dissolve the sugar in 2 tbsp water. Boil quickly until it is a dark brown liquid. Add a little water and heat gently until the caramel dissolves. Then add enough water to make a thin syrup. Bring to the boil, cool and bottle.

Only a small amount is needed to add colour to gravies.

Tahini gravy

Makes about 300 ml/½ pint

1 tbsp oil   *1 tsp brown rice miso, mixed to a thick*
1 tbsp rice flour   *paste with a little water*
1½ tsp tahini

Heat the oil in a pan. Add rice flour and tahini. Mix until a thick paste is formed. Slowly add 300 ml/½ pint water and miso and stir until a thick brown gravy is formed. A little homemade gravy browning (see above) can be added to give a richer colour.

Good with vegetarian dishes.

Coating batter

Makes about 150 ml/¼ pint

(1)

120 g/4 oz rice flour   *150 ml/¼ pint milk substitute*
⅛ tsp sea salt   *1 tsp commercial wheat-free baking*
1 tbsp Tomor margarine melted in a   *powder (see page 89)*
saucepan or 1 tbsp oil

Sift flour and salt together. Mix to a smooth consistency with the margarine or oil and milk and beat well.

Leave to stand for 30 minutes before using.

Just before using stir in the baking powder.

(2)

120 g/4 oz rice flour   *1 egg*
⅛ tsp salt   *150 ml/¼ pint milk substitute*

Turkey with apple and cherries (*bottom*, see page 78), Tossed green salad
OVERLEAF: Strawberry ice (*top left*, see page 106), Rhubarb fool (*top right*, see page 106), Apricot mould (*bottom left*, see page 106), Gingered-up pears (*bottom right*, see page 109)

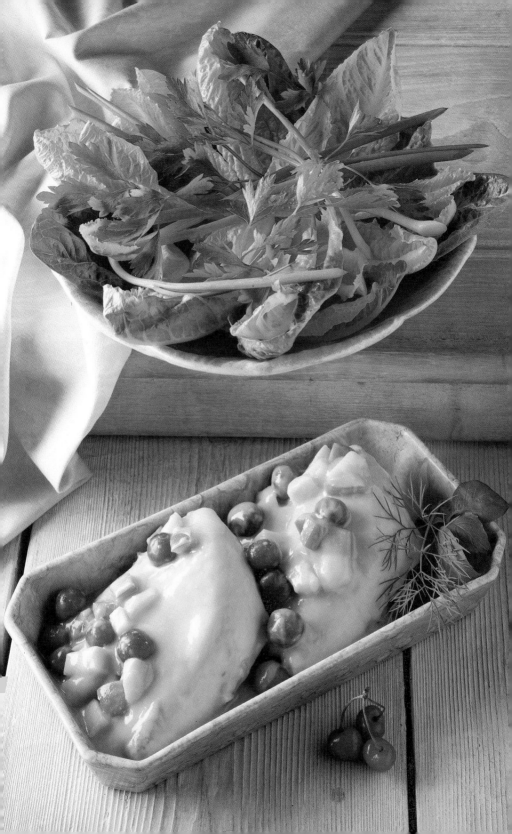

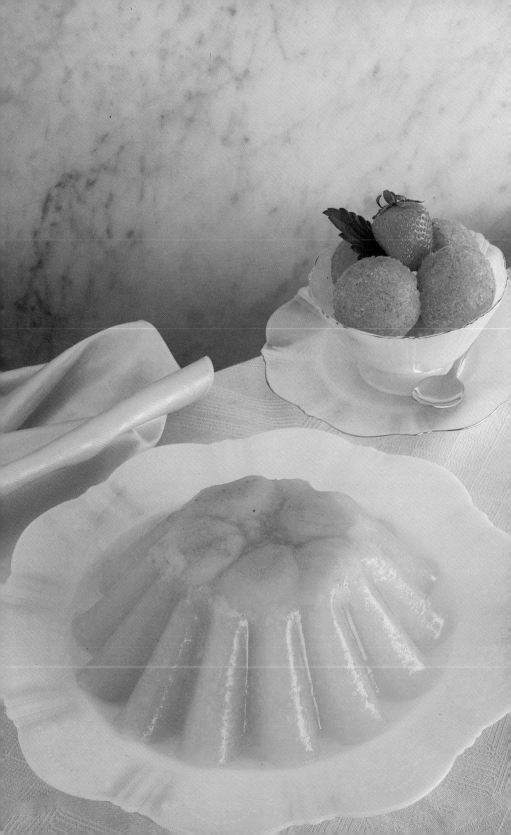

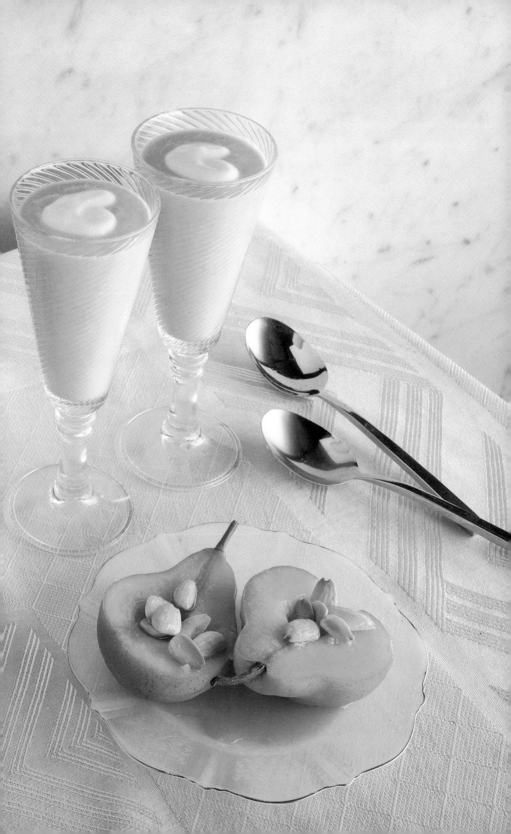

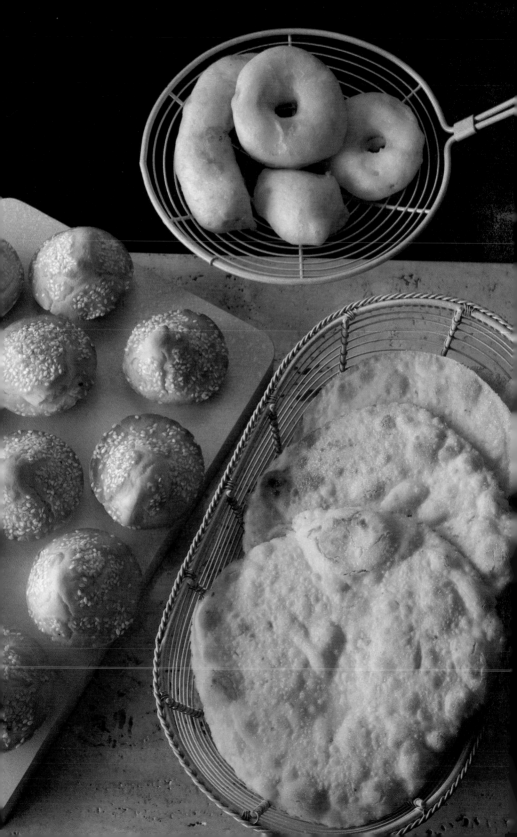

Sift flour and salt together. Make a well in the centre of the flour and add the egg and milk. Mix to a smooth consistency and beat well.
Leave to stand for 30 minutes before using.

Suggestions for use Coating for fried fish, fritters made with apple, banana or pineapple.

NB An excellent batter can also be made using gram flour; see recipe for pakoras (page 59) – spices can be omitted.

Basic white sauce

Makes about 60 ml/2 fl oz

15 g/½ oz Tomor margarine
15 g/½ oz soya flour

60–90 ml/2–3 fl oz milk substitute
salt and pepper

Melt the Tomor over low heat, add the flour and stir well. Let the mixture cook slowly for 2 minutes. Then gradually add the warmed milk substitute stirring all the time to prevent lumps and let it simmer gently for 2 minutes (if the sauce is too thick, add a little extra milk substitute). Add salt and pepper, stir well and serve.

Basic tomato sauce

Makes about 350 g/12 oz

450 g/1 lb tomatoes
1 tbsp oil (olive, sunflower, saf-flower, soya)

1 clove garlic, crushed
basil to taste
salt and pepper

Pour boiling water over the tomatoes, then drain after 1 minute. Plunge into cold water, drain and peel. Chop the tomatoes and place in a saucepan with oil, garlic, basil and seasoning. Simmer gently for 15 minutes.
Allow to cool and liquidize.
Reheat before serving.
This sauce is good with lamb, minced beef, pasta dishes, pizza, vegetables and pulses. It may be frozen.

Fruit fritters (bananas, pineapple, apple, *top*), Gram flour flatbread (*bottom right*, see page 91), Bread rolls (*bottom left*, see page 91)

Tomato ketchup   ✚ W M E

Serves 8

3 tbsp concentrated tomato purée
3 tbsp apple juice
1 tbsp gram flour

1 tbsp sunflower oil
salt and pepper
⅛ tsp chilli powder

Mix all ingredients together and season.

Raita   W M E

Serves 4   See photograph, page 54

450 ml/¾ pint yoghurt – goat's or
  ewe's
2 medium onions, finely chopped or
  half a cucumber, diced

2 tbsp chopped mint
⅛ tsp ground cumin
⅛ tsp chilli
salt and freshly ground black pepper

Beat all the ingredients together to make a smooth, creamy texture. If liked, crushed garlic may also be added.
   Serve with Indian dishes such as pakoras and gram flour flat bread.

Eggless mayonnaise   W M E

Makes about 250 ml/8 fl oz

½ tsp sea salt
1 tsp caster sugar
1 tsp dry mustard – wheat-free
pepper
1 tbsp rice flour

1 tsp arrowroot
4 tbsp oil (sunflower, safflower,
  olive, soya)
4 tbsp vinegar
200 ml/7 fl oz milk substitute

Mix salt, sugar, mustard, pepper and flours in a saucepan. Stir in oil. Add the vinegar gradually and lastly the milk substitute. Bring to the boil stirring all the time and cook until the sauce has thickened. Adjust seasoning when cold.

Salad dressing   ✚ W M E

Combine equal quantities of apple juice and olive oil. Beat to an emulsion, add a few grains of white sugar and salt and pepper to taste.

Yoghurt salad dressing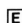

Makes about 150 ml/¼ pint

150 ml/¼ pint natural yoghurt –
  goat's or ewe's
1 tbsp chopped mint or chives

1 clove garlic, crushed
sea salt
pepper

Mix all the ingredients together just before serving.

Yoghurt curd cheese salad dressing

Serves 1

2 tsp sheep's yoghurt curd cheese
2 tsp sunflower oil

salt and pepper
mixed herbs to taste

Mix the curd cheese into the oil with the back of a spoon. Add the seasoning and herbs, then dilute with water to suit your taste. Use immediately.

Cheesy salad dressing

Serves 1

15 g/½ oz feta cheese
2 tsp sunflower oil
2 tsp apple juice

salt and pepper
chopped chives

Mix the cheese and oil to a paste with the back of a spoon. Stir in the apple juice, seasoning and herbs.
  Use immediately to toss a green salad.

Tahini salad dressing

Makes about 120 ml/4 fl oz

1½ tsp tahini
60 ml/2 fl oz oil
1 clove garlic, crushed
½ tsp basil
½ tsp sugar

½ tsp crushed mustard seeds
brown rice miso to taste – about ½ tsp
  mixed to a thick paste with a
  little water

Place the first six ingredients in a jug and stir well. Add miso and stir again.

BREAD AND PASTRY

Breadmaking

Many people using this book will have to eat wheat-free bread. This is more difficult to make than ordinary bread at first, and a few notes of warning are needed. However, there are a lot of tasty wheat-free loaves that can be successfully made with practice. We include a few in this book which we think are well worth the effort.

Yeast This can be bought either fresh or dried. Fresh yeast, wrapped in polythene or foil, will keep for four to five days in a cold place, a month in a refrigerator or a year in a deep-freeze. Dried yeast will keep up to six months if stored in a cool place. Half the amount of dried yeast is needed to fresh yeast, so, if 30 g/ 1 oz of fresh yeast is needed, use 15 g/½ oz of dried yeast. Temperature is very important when making yeast mixtures. Warm liquid accelerates the rising process, but if boiling liquids are used the yeast will be killed, and cold liquid slows growth.

Rising or proving time This depends on the temperature of the mixture. It may take forty-five to sixty minutes in a warm place such as an airing cupboard, two hours at room temperature. It is therefore better to go by the look of the mixture than try to time it. The mixture should double in volume before baking.

Dough Wheat-free breads will form a batter or cake-like consistency when mixed rather than an ordinary dough. This is because the flours used lack gluten, the protein that provides the elasticity and structure in ordinary bread.

Baking Bread is baked in a very hot oven 230 °C/450 °F/gas 8 to kill the yeast. Loaf tins should only be half filled with the dough to allow space for rising. When baked the crust will be a golden brown colour. Allow the bread to cool slightly before turning out of the baking tin.

Storage Wheat-free breads tend to dry out quickly. Therefore store in a plastic bag for short periods or in a freezer for long storage. If the bread is sliced before freezing a few slices can be taken out and thawed when needed.

Baking powder

Baking powder contains starch such as rice flour, cornflour and frequently wheat flour. Always check the list of ingredients on any bought baking powder to make sure it is safe for you. Commercial wheat-free brands currently available in the UK are the Co-op's and Sainsbury's, and from health food shops, Bestoval, Food Watch, Hinton and Rite-Diet. If you are unable to find a suitable baking powder you can make your own:

Homemade wheat-free baking powder

60 g/2 oz rice flour　　　　　　*130 g/4½ oz cream of tartar*
60 g/2 oz bicarbonate of soda

Sieve the ingredients together at least 3 times. Store in an airtight container in a dry place.

NB The recipes in this book are made with commercial wheat-free baking powder. If using homemade, slightly more is required, eg, if 2 tsp baking powder is stated in the recipe, use 3 tsp homemade powder.

Rusks　　　　　　　　　　　　　

Wheat-free bread　　　　　　　*2 tbsp honey*
300 ml/½ pint milk substitute

Cut wheat-free bread into slices about 1 cm/½ in thick. Cut these into fingers and dip into a mixture of milk substitute and honey.
　　Bake in a medium oven until dry.
　　Cool and store in an airtight container. This is a good way of using up stale bread.

Plain white bread　　　　

Makes 1 × 900 g/2 lb loaf

30 g/1 oz fresh yeast or 15 g/½ oz　*60 g/2 oz soya flour*
*　dried yeast*　　　　　　　　　　*120 g/4 oz rice flour*
1 tsp sugar　　　　　　　　　　　*1 tsp salt*
30 g/1 oz Tomor margarine　　　*240 ml/8 fl oz milk substitute*
170 g/6 oz millet flour

See breadmaking notes opposite.
　　Sprinkle the yeast on a mixture of 90 ml/3 fl oz warm water and sugar. Allow to stand until the liquid froths, about 10–20 minutes.

Add the Tomor cut into small pieces, then the sifted flours, salt and milk substitute. Beat until the mixture is smooth and creamy. Put the bowl in a plastic bag and allow to prove in a warm place.

Preheat oven to 230 °C/450 °F/gas 8. Pour mixture into a well greased 900 g/2 lb loaf tin and bake for 30 minutes.

Brown bread

Makes 1 × 900 g/2 lb loaf

*30 g/1 oz fresh yeast or 15 g/½ oz
dried yeast
1 tsp sugar
30 g/1 oz Tomor margarine
170 g/6 oz buckwheat flour*

*170 g/6 oz potato flour
1 tsp carob flour
1 tsp salt
180 ml/6 fl oz milk substitute
1 egg*

See breadmaking notes (page 88).

Sprinkle the yeast on to 90 ml/3 fl oz warm water and sugar. Allow to stand until the mixture froths, about 10–20 minutes.

Add the Tomor cut into small pieces then the sifted flours, salt, milk substitute and egg. Beat until the mixture is smooth. Put the bowl in a plastic bag and allow to prove in a warm place.

Preheat oven to 230 °C/450 °F/Gas 8. Pour mixture into a well greased 900 g/2 lb loaf tin and bake for 30 minutes.

Potato and rice flour bread

Makes 1 × 450 g/1 lb loaf

*15 g/½ oz fresh yeast or 7 g/¼ oz dried
yeast
½ tsp sugar
85 g/3 oz potato flour*

*85 g/3 oz rice flour
½ tsp salt
15 g/½ oz Tomor margarine*

See breadmaking notes (page 88).

Mix yeast with sugar and 180 ml/6 fl oz warm water. Leave to froth for 10–20 minutes. Sift the flours and salt together. Add margarine cut into small pieces and yeast mixture. Beat well. Put bowl in a plastic bag and leave to prove in a warm place.

Preheat oven to 230 °C/450 °F/gas 8. Pour mixture into a greased 450 g/1 lb loaf tin and bake for 30 minutes.

An alternative   For a wheat-free and milk-free loaf, reduce the water to 150 ml/¼ pint and add 1 egg to the flour at the same time as the yeast mixture.

Bread rolls

Makes 9 small rolls See photograph, page 84

15 g/½ oz fresh yeast or 7 g/¼ oz dried   *60 g/2 oz rice flour*
    yeast   *60 g/2 oz soya flour*
½ tsp sugar   *½ tsp salt*
15 g/½ oz Tomor margarine   *1 egg*
60 g/2 oz potato flour   *sesame seeds*

See breadmaking notes (page 88).

Sprinkle the yeast on to 150 ml/5 fl oz warm water and sugar mixture. Allow to stand and froth for about 10–20 minutes.

Add the Tomor cut into small pieces, the sifted flours, salt and egg. Beat until the mixture is smooth and creamy. Put the bowl in a plastic bag and leave to prove in a warm place.

Preheat oven to 230 °C/450 °F/gas 8. Spoon the dough into greased bun tins and sprinkle with sesame seeds. Bake for 15 minutes.

Rice loaf

Makes 1 × 900 g/2 lb loaf

150 ml/5 fl oz sunflower, safflower or   *250 g/9 oz rice flour*
    soya oil   *2 tsp commercial wheat-free baking*
170 g/6 oz caster sugar   *powder (see page 89)*
3 large beaten eggs   *1–2 tbsp milk substitute*

Preheat oven to 180 °C/350 °F/gas 4.

Grease a 900 g/2 lb loaf tin.

Beat oil and sugar together. Add the beaten egg a little at a time. Beat in sifted flour and baking powder. Add milk substitute to give a dropping consistency and beat well.

Pour into prepared tin and bake for 1–1½ hours.

Leave in tin until cool and then turn out.

Gram flour flatbread

Makes 4–6 See photograph, page 84

2 tsp oil + oil for frying   *⅛ tsp chilli powder (or to taste)*
120 g/4 oz gram flour   *1 tsp cumin*
¼ tsp salt   or
a little rice flour   *any selection of chopped mixed fresh*
and either   *herbs, eg, parsley, chives*

Rub 2 tsp oil into flour. Add salt and spices or herbs. Work into a dough with approximately 60 ml/2 fl oz water. Make into 4 or 6

balls. Roll out into flat circles on a board floured with rice flour.
Fry in a little oil until brown on both sides.
Serve hot.

Fruit scones

Makes 12–15

225 g/8 oz sago or rice flour
2 tsp commercial wheat-free baking
powder (see page 89)
60 g/2 oz Tomor margarine

60 g/2 oz sugar
60 g/2 oz dried fruit
1 egg
60 ml/2 fl oz milk substitute

Preheat oven to 230 °C/450 °F/gas 8.
Sift flour and baking powder together and rub in Tomor. Add the sugar and dried fruit and mix together to a soft dough with the lightly beaten egg and milk.
Drop the mixture with a dessert spoon on to a greased baking sheet. Brush lightly with beaten egg or milk and bake for 15–20 minutes.

Apple and walnut tea bread

Makes 1 × 900 g/2 lb loaf

120 g/4 oz potato flour
120 g/4 oz rice flour
1 tsp commercial wheat-free baking
powder (see page 89)
⅛ tsp salt
1 level tsp mixed spices
120 g/4 oz Tomor margarine

120 g/4 oz caster sugar
2 large eggs
1 tbsp golden syrup or honey
120 g/4 oz sultanas
60 g/2 oz well chopped walnuts
1 cooking apple, peeled, cored and chopped

Preheat oven to 160 °C/325 °F/gas 3.
Grease a 900 g/2 lb loaf tin and line the base with greased paper.
Sieve flours, baking powder, salt and mixed spices.
Cream Tomor and sugar together. Beat in 1 egg, syrup and 1 tbsp mixed flours. Beat in second egg and stir in the remainder of the flour, fruit, walnuts and apple. Put mixture in tin and level it. Bake for 1–1½ hours.
Turn out when cool and dredge with icing sugar.

Apple and walnut teabread (*top*), Pear and carob cake (*centre left*, see page 99), Plum bake (*centre right*, see page 96)

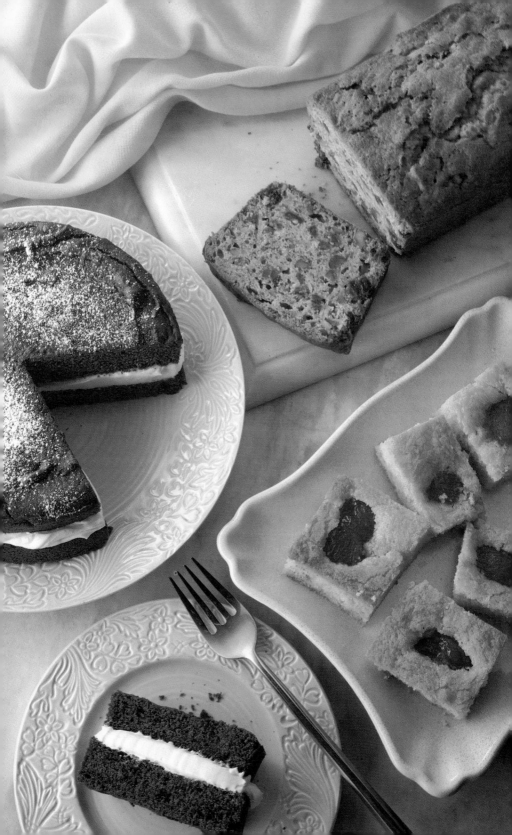

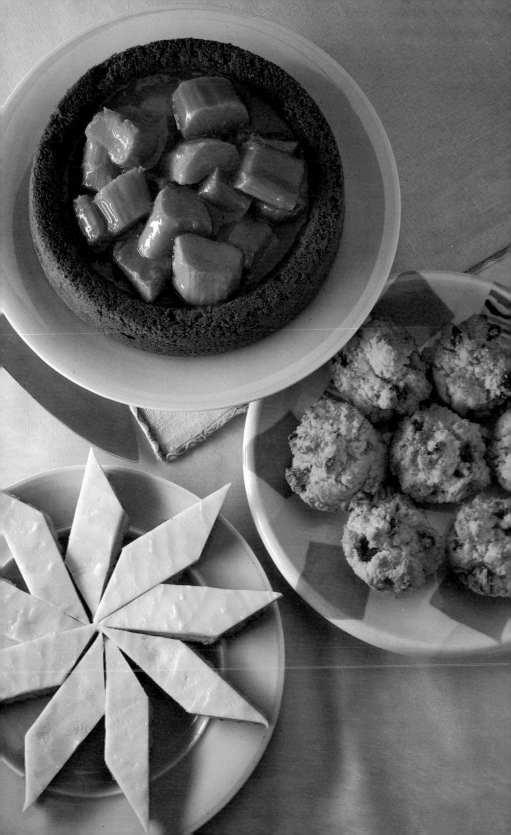

Savoury shortcrust pastry ☒ Ⓦ Ⓜ Ⓔ

To cover 1 × 18 cm/7 in pie dish

120 g/4 oz gram flour   *60 g/2 oz Tomor margarine*
⅛ tsp salt

Mix the flour and salt together. Cut the margarine into small pieces and rub it in to the flour until the mixture resembles fine breadcrumbs. Mix in water with a round-bladed knife until the mixture begins to stick together. Collect the mixture together with one hand, and knead lightly for a few seconds.
    Roll out the dough in one direction only, on a floured surface, using gram flour.
    Bake for 15–20 minutes at 220 °C/425 °F/gas 7.
    Use as required.

Sweet shortcrust pastry ☒ Ⓦ Ⓜ Ⓔ

To cover 1 × 18 cm/7 in pie dish

120 g/4 oz gram flour   *60 g/2 oz Tomor margarine*
60 g/2 oz caster sugar

Sieve together the dry ingredients and rub in the Tomor. Gradually stir in about 4 tsp cold water to produce a suitable consistency for rolling out.
    Bake for 15–20 minutes at 220 °C/425 °F/gas 7.
    Use as required.

Buckwheat pastry ☒ Ⓦ Ⓜ Ⓔ

To cover 2 × 18 cm/7 in pie dishes

150 g/5 oz Tomor margarine   *120 g/4 oz rice flour*
⅛ tsp salt   *1 tsp cream of tartar*
120 g/4 oz buckwheat flour   *½ tsp bicarbonate of soda*

Use margarine straight from the refrigerator. Cream the margarine, 1–1½ tsp water, salt and one-third of the sifted flours in a mixing bowl. Mix in the remaining flour, cream of tartar and bicarbonate of soda and knead until smooth, adding more water if necessary. Roll out thinly on a floured surface, using rice flour.
    Bake for 20 minutes at 220 °C/425 °F/gas 7.
    Good with both sweet and savoury pie fillings.

Fruit flan (*top*, see page 107), Millet and date buns (*centre*, see page 100), Crunchy ginger slices (*bottom*, see page 102)

CAKES AND BISCUITS

Plum bake

Serves 4   See photograph, page 93

120 g/4 oz Tomor margarine
100 g/3½ oz caster sugar
1 medium size egg
30 g/1 oz potato flour
60 g/2 oz ground rice

30 g/1 oz soya flour
½ tsp commercial wheat-free baking
   powder (see page 89)
8 plums

Preheat oven to 180 °C/350 °F/gas 4.

Cream the Tomor and 85 g/3 oz caster sugar together. Beat in the egg. Stir in the sifted flours and baking powder. Spread the mixture on to a greased 18 cm/7 in square tin.

Halve and stone the plums and press the halves into the surface of the mixture. Sprinkle with the remaining caster sugar.

Bake for 35–40 minutes or until firm when pressed in centre.

Cut into squares when hot and serve as a pudding with goat's or ewe's yoghurt, or serve it cold as cake.

An alternative Dried apricots (soaked and cooked) can be substituted for plums.

Spicy honeycake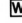

85 g/3 oz clear honey
120 g/4 oz rice flour
60 g/2 oz potato flour
60 g/2 oz soya flour
1 level tsp ground ginger
1 level tsp ground cinnamon
¼ tsp ground cloves
85 g/3 oz caster sugar
finely grated rind of 1 small orange
finely grated rind of 1 small lemon
120 g/4 oz Tomor margarine

1 large egg, beaten
1 level tsp bicarbonate of soda, dissolved in 3 tbsp water
60 g/2 oz mixed candied peel, finely
   chopped

Icing:
120 g/4 oz icing sugar
1½ tbsp lemon juice
2 tbsp warm water

Preheat oven to 160 °C/325 °F/gas 3.

Weigh a cup on the scales and then weigh honey in it. Place the cup in a saucepan containing simmering water and warm the honey a little.

Sift the flours and spices into a large mixing bowl, then add sugar and the orange and lemon rinds. Add the Tomor in small pieces and rub it into the flours until it resembles fine breadcrumbs. Mix in the beaten egg using a large fork, and then add the honey. Add the bicarbonate of soda in water to cake mixture. Beat hard until the mixture is smooth and soft.

Stir in the mixed peel and spoon the mixture into a 18 cm/7 in square greased tin. Bake for 45 minutes. Cool before turning out on to a wire rack.

Make up the icing and spread it over the cooled cake.

Sponge cake

3 eggs
85 g/3 oz caster sugar
85 g/3 oz sago flour
*1 tsp commercial wheat-free baking
  powder (see page 89)*

Fillings:
*stewed apple, nut cream (see page 110),
  jam or any other filling allowed*

Preheat oven to 180 °C/350 °F/gas 4.

Grease two 18 cm/7 in sandwich tins.

Put the eggs and sugar in a bowl over a pan of hot water. Beat until thick and creamy. Fold in sifted flour and baking powder. Divide the mixture between the tins and bake for 20 minutes until golden brown.

When cold sandwich together with chosen filling.

An alternative   Rice flour can be substituted for sago flour.

Gingerbread

170 g/6 oz rice flour
2 tsp ground ginger
1 tsp mixed spice
½ tsp bicarbonate of soda
*1½ tsp commercial wheat-free baking
  powder (see page 89)*
120 ml/4 fl oz golden syrup

*30 ml/1 fl oz sunflower, safflower or
  soya oil*
30 g/1 oz caster sugar
2 tbsp milk substitute
1 level tbsp black treacle
1 beaten egg

Preheat oven to 180 °C/350 °F/gas 4.

Sift the flour, ginger, mixed spice, bicarbonate of soda and baking powder into a bowl. Make a well in the centre. Melt the syrup, oil and sugar in a pan over a low heat. Pour on to the flour mixture. Add milk, treacle and egg. Beat until smooth. Pour into a greased 15 cm/6 in tin. Bake for 1 hour.

Turn out on to a wire rack and cool.

Ground rice cake

120 g/4 oz Tomor margarine
120 g/4 oz caster sugar
2 eggs
120 g/4 oz ground rice
60 g/2 oz potato flour

grated rind of 1 lemon
juice of ½ lemon
½ tsp bicarbonate of soda stirred into 1
   tsp milk substitute

Preheat oven to 180 °C/350 °F/gas 4.
   Cream the Tomor and sugar together. Add 1 egg. Combine the
flours and stir in 1 tsp of flour mixture. Add the second egg and
rind of lemon and mix. Add remainder of flour and juice of lemon.
Mix well with the bicarbonate of soda in milk substitute.
   Place in a greased 18 cm/7 in cake tin and bake for 1½
hours.

Snow cake

120 g/4 oz Tomor margarine
120 g/4 oz caster sugar
2 eggs

225 g/8 oz potato flour
1 tsp commercial wheat-free baking
   powder (see page 89)

Preheat oven to 160 °C/325 °F/gas 3.
   Cream Tomor and sugar together. Add eggs and potato flour.
Stir in the baking powder. Beat for 10 minutes.
   Pour into a flat 18 × 28 cm/7 × 11 in baking tin, greased and
lightly floured. The mixture should cover the tin to a depth of
about 1 cm/½ in. Bake for 30 minutes.
   Turn out when cold. Cover with icing (lemon-flavoured is very
good), and cut into finger lengths.

Buckwheat cake

150 ml/5 fl oz runny honey
150 ml/5 fl oz sunflower oil
2 eggs

170 g/6 oz buckwheat flour
4½ tsp commercial wheat-free baking
   powder (see page 89)

Preheat oven to 160 °C/325 °F/gas 3.
   Grease and flour an 18 cm/7 in cake tin.
   Beat together honey, oil and eggs. Sift together flour and bak-
ing powder at least twice. Beat the dry ingredients into the first
mixture. Pour the mixture into prepared cake tin.
   Bake for 50–60 minutes.

Carob cake   W M

150 ml/5 fl oz runny honey
150 ml/5 fl oz sunflower oil
2 eggs

170 g/6 oz carob flour
4½ tsp commercial wheat-free baking
   powder (see page 89)

Preheat oven to 160 °C/325 °F/gas 3.

Beat together the honey, oil and eggs. Sift together flour and baking powder at least twice. Beat the dry ingredients into the wet ones.

Put into 2 prepared 18 cm/7 in cake tins. Bake for 1 hour.

Allow to cool, and sandwich together either with icing sugar creamed with Tomor, and softened with a little milk substitute if necessary, or with homemade or preservative-free commercial jam.

Buckwheat fruit cake

[✶] [W] [M] [E]

120 g/4 oz rice flour
120 g/4 oz buckwheat flour
120 g/4 oz Tomor margarine
120 g/4 oz brown sugar
2 tsp commercial wheat-free baking powder (see page 89)
120 g/4 oz sultanas and currants mixed
60 g/2 oz chopped dates
milk substitute to mix

Preheat oven to 180 °C/350 °F/gas 4.

Sift flours into a bowl. Rub in Tomor until it resembles fine breadcrumbs. Add sugar, baking powder and dried fruit and enough milk substitute to give a stiff consistency.

Put into a greased 15 cm/6 in cake tin. Bake for 1 hour.

An alternative Can be made entirely with rice flour.

Pear and carob cake

[✶] [W] [M] [E]

see photograph, page 93

120 g/4 oz Tomor margarine
150 g/5 oz rice flour
30 g/1 oz carob flour
85 g/3 oz soya flour
120 g/4 oz brown sugar
2 pears, stewed, cooled and liquidized
1–2 tbsp milk substitute
1 level tsp sodium bicarbonate in 2 tsp water

Filling:
60 g/2 oz Tomor margarine
85 g/3 oz icing sugar

Preheat oven to 180 °C/350 °F/gas 4.

Rub Tomor into flours, then add sugar. Mix thoroughly. Make a well in centre and slowly stir in pears and milk substitute until all the flour has been taken up. the mixture should be slightly sloppy. Add bicarbonate of soda. Beat the mixture hard until it becomes smooth and fluffy. This is important: if the beating does not reach this stage the cake will be flat and unpalatable.

Turn immediately into two 18 cm/7 in greased cake tins. Bake for 25–30 minutes.

For the filling cream the Tomor, add sugar gradually and beat together. When the cake is cool, sandwich the two halves together with the filling.

Apple cake ⊞W ⊞M

450 g/1 lb cooking apples
170 g/6 oz Tomor margarine
225 g/8 oz caster sugar
2 large eggs
120 g/4 oz potato flour
60 g/2 oz rice flour

60 g/2 oz soya flour
2 tsp commercial wheat-free baking
　powder (see page 89)
⅛ tsp salt
ground cinnamon to taste

Preheat oven to 180 °C/350 °F/gas 4.

Peel, core and cut apples into slices. Cook very gently in 30 g/1 oz Tomor until apple is approximately half cooked. Remove from heat.

Cream rest of Tomor and sugar together. Beat the eggs into the mixture. Fold in the sifted flours, baking powder and salt. Put half the cake mixture into a greased cake tin 23 cm/9 in in diameter. Arrange the apple slices over this and sprinkle with cinnamon. Cover with the remaining cake mixture. Bake for 1½ hours.

Cool slightly before removing from the tin. Dust with icing sugar when completely cool.

Millet and date buns ⊞W ⊞M

Makes 12–16 buns　　　　　See photograph, page 94

225 g/8 oz millet flour
4 tsp commercial wheat-free baking
　powder (see page 89)
60 g/2 oz Tomor margarine

60 ml/2 fl oz milk substitute
2 eggs
60 g/2 oz sugar
120 g/4 oz dates, chopped

Preheat oven to 220 °C/425 °F/gas 7.

Sift flour and baking powder together; rub in Tomor. Mix milk substitute, eggs, sugar and dates together and add to the flour. Beat to a stiff consistency. Spoon into greased bun tins or paper cases. Bake for 15–20 minutes.

Alternatives　Omit dates and add any one of the following.
Carob buns: use 200 g/7 oz millet flour and 30 g/1 oz carob
　flour.
Coconut buns: add 60 g/2 oz desiccated coconut to the mixture.
Ginger buns: add 2 tsp ground ginger to the flour.
Seed buns: add 1½ tsp caraway seeds to the mixture.

Rice Krispie cakes ⊞★ ⊞W ⊞M ⊞E

Makes 20–24 cakes

2 tbsp honey or golden syrup
30 g/1 oz brown sugar

at least 30 g/1 oz Rice Krispies

Heat honey and sugar until sugar dissolves. Stir in enough Rice Krispies to absorb the honey. Spoon into paper cases and leave to cool and harden.

Alternatives Chopped dates or 2 tsp carob flour may be added.

Savoury buckwheat biscuits

Makes 8–10 biscuits

100 g/3½ oz buckwheat flour
⅛ tsp salt
1½ tsp commercial wheat-free baking
powder (see page 89)

30 g/1 oz Tomor margarine
60 ml/2 fl oz milk substitute

Preheat oven to 190 °C/375 °F/gas 5.

Sift together flour, salt and baking powder at least twice. Rub in the Tomor. Make a well in the centre and gradually pour in the milk, stirring to form a soft dough.

Turn on to a floured board and roll out to 1 cm/½ in thick. Cut into rounds, arrange on a greased baking sheet and bake for 10–15 minutes.

These are good to use in packed lunches.

Buckwheat and rice crackers

Makes 15–20 biscuits

150 g/5 oz Tomor margarine
120 g/4 oz rice flour
120 g/4 oz buckwheat flour

⅛ tsp salt
1 tsp cream of tartar
½ tsp bicarbonate of soda

Preheat oven to 180 °C/350 °F/gas 4.

In a mixing bowl cream the Tomor with 1–1½ tsp water, salt and one-third of the flours (for best results use margarine straight from the refrigerator). Mix in the remaining flour, cream of tartar and bicarbonate of soda until smooth. Add more water if necessary to make a soft dough.

Roll out the dough thinly on a floured surface. Cut into squares and place on a greased baking sheet. Bake for about ½ hour until brown.

These are very good with goat's cheese.

Shortbread

Makes 8–10 pieces

85 g/3 oz soya flour
85 g/3 oz rice flour
60 g/2 oz caster or granulated sugar

100 g/3½ oz Tomor margarine
30 ml/1 fl oz milk substitute

Preheat oven to 160 °C/325 °F/gas 3.
Grease and flour a 18 cm/7 in square or circular shallow tin.
Sift together the soya and rice flours, then sift with the sugar.
Rub in the Tomor and stir in the milk substitute. Mix lightly to
form a dough and press into the tin to a thickness of about 1 cm/½
in. Prick surface with a fork.
Bake for 45 minutes.

Chestnut shortbread   🗙 Ⓦ Ⓜ Ⓔ

Makes 10–15 pieces

60 g/2 oz chestnut flour
85 g/3 oz ground rice
grated rind of 1 lemon

cinnamon or mixed spice to taste
1½ tsp fructose
1 tbsp safflower oil

Preheat oven to 180 °C/350 °F/gas 4.
Mix all the ingredients together and rub in the oil with finger-
tips. Gather lightly to form a dough and press into a greased 20
cm/8 in square or circular shallow tin to a thickness of about
1 cm/½ in. Prick the surface and bake for 20 minutes.

Iced gingernuts   🗙 Ⓦ Ⓜ Ⓔ

Makes 12–16

30 g/1 oz Tomor margarine
30 g/1 oz soft brown sugar
60 g/2 oz golden syrup
60 g/2 oz soya flour
30 g/1 oz rice flour

1 tsp commercial wheat-free baking
powder (see page 89)
½ tsp cream of tartar
½ tsp ground ginger
glacé icing

Preheat oven to 180 °C/350 °F/gas 4.
Melt the Tomor in a pan on low heat and stir in the golden syrup
and sugar. Sift together the dry ingredients and then re-sift them
into the pan. Stir to a firm paste. Take small spoonfuls and roll in
the hands until smooth (walnut size), then flatten on a greased
baking tray. Bake for 15–17 minutes.
Leave to cool, then decorate with glacé icing.

Crunchy ginger slices   🗙 Ⓦ Ⓜ Ⓔ

120 g/4 oz Tomor margarine
120 g/4 oz sugar
60 g/2 oz soya flour
150 g/5 oz potato flour
1 tsp ground ginger
1 tsp commercial wheat-free baking
powder (see page 89)

Icing:
60 g/2 oz Tomor margarine
170 g/6 oz icing sugar
2 tsp ground ginger
4 tsp honey

(see photograph, page 94)

Preheat oven to 190 °C/375 °F/gas 5.

Cream Tomor and sugar together. Add sifted flours, ginger and baking powder. Knead well.

Roll flat and press into a greased shallow tin 23 cm × 28 cm/9 in × 11 in.

Bake for 25 minutes and allow to cool.

To make the icing, melt all the ingredients in a saucepan. Spread on to the biscuit with a wetted, round-bladed knife. Cut into slices before the icing is completely cold.

Currant cookies

Makes about 16

30 g/1 oz Tomor margarine
30 g/1 oz pale demerara sugar
2 tbsp golden syrup
120 g/4 oz rice flour

1 tsp commercial wheat-free baking
powder (see page 89)
1 tsp cream of tartar
30 g/1 oz currants

Preheat oven to 180 °C/350 °F/gas 4.

Melt Tomor in a pan over a low heat and stir in sugar and golden syrup until dissolved. Combine dry ingredients and sift into pan. Mix to a firm paste, with the currants evenly distributed. Take small spoonfuls and roll until smooth – about the size of a whole walnut. Flatten and place well apart on a greased baking tin.

Cook for 15–20 minutes and cool on baking sheet.

Best eaten within 48 hours.

Millet flake flapjacks

120 g/4 oz Tomor margarine
60 g/2 oz demerara sugar

1 tbsp runny honey
170 g/6 oz millet flakes

Preheat oven to 180 °C/350 °F/gas 4.

Cream the margarine and sugar. Add the honey and millet flakes. Mix well.

Press into a greased baking tray 20 cm/8 in square. Bake for 15 minutes.

Mark into squares and allow to cool before lifting off the tray.

Rice Krispie cookies ⊞ ⊞

Makes 12–16 small biscuits

45 g/1½ oz Rice Krispies
2 egg whites
1½ tsp clear honey

60 g/2 oz caster sugar
rice paper

Preheat oven to 190 °C/375 °F/gas 5.
Spread rice paper on a baking sheet.
Crush the Rice Krispies with a rolling pin. Whisk egg whites until they are very stiff. Add honey and fold in sugar and Rice Krispies. Spoon on to rice paper. Bake for 20–25 minutes.

Carob biscuits

Makes 15–20 biscuits

120 g/4 oz Tomor margarine	30 g/1 oz carob flour
75 g/2½ oz caster sugar	2 tbsp oil
200 g/7 oz rice flour	1 egg

Preheat oven to 180 °C/350 °F/gas 4.
Cream Tomor and 60 g/2 oz sugar together. Work in the sieved flours, oil and egg and knead well.
Roll out to ½ cm/¼ in thick, and cut into shapes. Prick each biscuit with a fork and put on a baking tray, oiled and dusted with rice flour. Bake for about 15 minutes until firm and crisp. Dredge with remaining caster sugar while still warm.
Remove from tray when cold.

FRUIT AND PUDDINGS

Summer fruit dessert

Serves 4

1–2 nectarines	225 g/8 oz raspberries or strawberries
1–2 peaches	sugar to taste
225 g/8 oz red or black currants, topped and tailed	

Stew the currants in 2 tbsp water and sweeten to taste. Allow to cool.
Wash the nectarines and peaches and slice into quarters.
Wash the soft fruit.
Mix all together and chill before serving.
Shortbread is a good accompaniment to this pudding (see page 101).

Anytime-of-year fruit salad

Serves 4–6

½ pineapple
1–2 bananas
1 eating apple from each of the different varieties, eg, Cox's, Granny Smith's, Golden Delicious

120 g/4 oz fresh or frozen raspberries or strawberries
340 g/12 oz gooseberries, fresh or bottled
sugar (optional)

Cut the pineapple out of its jacket in coarse chunks. Be careful to cut out the eyes and to save all the juice for other dishes, or to drink. Skin and chop bananas. Core and slice apples. Mix all the fruits together and add sugar to taste if desired. Chill before serving.

Dried fruit compote

Serves 6

30 g/1 oz sugar
5–8 cm/2–3 in stick of cinnamon
450 g/1 lb mixed dried fruit, eg, apple

rings, peaches, apricots, prunes, pears and sultanas

Dissolve the sugar in 600 ml/1 pint water over a gentle heat. Add the cinnamon. Place the dried fruit in a bowl and pour over the syrup. Cover and leave to soak overnight.

If the soaked fruit is not tender, place in a pan and simmer for a few minutes.

Serve cold with yoghurt.

Fruit jelly

Serves 4

22 g/¾ oz gelatine
600 ml/1 pint unsweetened fruit juice,

eg, apple or pineapple

Sprinkle the gelatine on 90 ml/3 fl oz heated fruit juice, and stir well till dissolved. Add the rest of the juice. Put into a wetted mould and chill until set.

An alternative This can be made with sweetened milk substitute to give a milk jelly. Sprinkle the gelatine on to 4 tbsp water then heat gently to dissolve. Add the gelatine to 600 ml/1 pint milk substitute while still hot but not boiling. The milk substitute may be flavoured with vanilla if liked.

Strawberry ice   ⊠ Ⓦ Ⓜ Ⓔ

Serves 4–6   See photograph, page 82

280 g/10 oz strawberries, fresh or   *30 g/1 oz sugar*
frozen   *15 g/½ oz powdered gelatine*

Liquidize the strawberries and sugar together. Dissolve the gelatine in 250 ml/8 fl oz warm water. Mix with the fruit. Put in a freezer or freezer compartment of the refrigerator. When partially frozen, beat well, if possible with an electric beater, then freeze until firm.

Rhubarb fool   ⊠ Ⓦ Ⓜ Ⓔ

Serves 2   See photograph, page 83

30 g/1 oz Tomor margarine   *30 g/1 oz brown sugar*
225 g/½ lb rhubarb   *200 ml/7 oz goat's or ewe's yoghurt*

Melt the Tomor in a pan. Add the rhubarb and sugar and cook until tender. Liquidize rhubarb and yoghurt together.
Chill before serving.

Apricot mould   ⊠ Ⓦ Ⓜ Ⓔ

Serves 4   See photograph, page 82

130 g/4½ oz dried apricots   *1 sachet powdered gelatine (about*
2 tbsp granulated sugar   *15 g/½ oz)*

Pour boiling water over 100 g/3½ oz apricots and leave to soak for several hours. Drain and wash. Stew for 10 minutes until soft in 60 ml/2 fl oz water. Sieve to make a purée, then stir in the sugar.
    Dissolve the gelatine in 90 ml/3 fl oz very hot water, stirring briskly. Make up to 300 ml/½ pint with cold water, then stir into the apricot mixture.
    Arrange the remaining dried apricots on the base of a wetted mould, then carefully pour the mixture in. Set in a refrigerator for 3 hours.

Grantchester dessert   Ⓦ Ⓜ Ⓔ

Serves 1

1 tbsp honey   *sprinkling of chopped almonds*
100 g/3½ oz sheep's yoghurt   *or fresh fruit*

Spoon the honey into the bottom of a ramekin and add the yoghurt on top. Garnish with nuts or fruit.
    This is portable, and so also good as part of a snack lunch.

Peach condé ☒ Ⓦ Ⓜ Ⓔ

Serves 6 | See photograph, page 111

60 g/2 oz short grain rice
600 ml/1 pint milk substitute
60 g/2 oz caster sugar

1 tin peaches (preservative-free) or 3
* fresh peaches*
30 g/1 oz arrowroot

Wash the rice and simmer with the milk substitute until thick and creamy. Leave to cool. Add sugar.

Divide rice between six serving dishes. If using tinned peaches, drain and put one peach half on each dish. Thicken the juice with arrowroot. If using fresh peaches, skin and halve and put one half on each dish. Make an arrowroot sauce with 300 ml/½ pint liquid, eg, apple juice. Pour the arrowroot sauce over the fruit and leave to set.

Rice flake mould ☒ Ⓦ Ⓜ Ⓔ

Serves 4

85 g/3 oz rice flakes
600 ml/1 pint milk substitute

45 g/1½ oz caster sugar

Sprinkle rice flakes into near boiling milk substitute and cover pan with lid. Simmer until tender (10–15 minutes) and the milk almost absorbed. Sweeten with the sugar. Pour quickly into a cold, wet basin or mould. Turn out when set, after about 2 hours.

Serve with stewed fruit.

Fruit flan ☒ Ⓦ Ⓜ Ⓔ

Serves 4–5 | See photograph, page 94

1 egg
75 ml/2½ fl oz clear honey
75 ml/2½ fl oz sunflower oil
85 g/3 oz buckwheat flour
2½ tsp commercial wheat-free baking
* powder (see page 89)*

350 g/12 oz rhubarb or other allowed
* fruit*
2–3 tbsp sugar
1 sachet powdered gelatine (about
* 15 g/½ oz)*
apple slices to garnish

Preheat oven to 160 °C/325 °F/gas 3.

Blend together the egg, honey and sunflower oil. Sieve in the buckwheat flour and baking powder. Mix well then pour into a greased 18 cm/7 in flan tin. Bake for 30–35 minutes.

Meanwhile, stew the rhubarb, or whatever fruit you are using, with the sugar in a minimum of water.

Mix the gelatine in 150 ml/¼ pint of very hot water. When it dissolves make up to 300 ml/½ pint with cold water. Stir in the rhubarb and juice and place in a bowl to set.

When almost set, pile on to the flan base and decorate with apple slices just before serving.

Crispy caramel fruit   ☒ Ⓦ Ⓜ Ⓔ

Serves 4

4 dessert apples   *halved pipped black grapes*
2 bananas   *enough demerara sugar to cover fruit*

Peel and core the apples and stew in a little water until soft. Mash if necessary, and spoon into ovenproof ramekins. Arrange sliced banana to cover as much as possible of the apple. Decorate with grape halves.

Sprinkle with sugar and place under a hot grill until the sugar has melted, or bake in a hot oven for 10 minutes.

Stuffed baked apples   ☒ Ⓦ Ⓜ Ⓔ

Serves 4

4 cooking apples   Stuffing:
1 tbsp honey   *dates, honey and ground cloves or*
                           cinnamon
                           or
                           raisins and brown sugar

Preheat oven to 200 °C/400 °F/gas 6.

Core the apples and slit the skin in a ring round the middle. Stuff with chosen filling and put in a baking dish.

Add 5 mm/¼ in of water and 1 tbsp of honey to the baking dish. Bake until the fruit is tender.

Serve hot or cold.

Baked bananas   ☒ Ⓦ Ⓜ Ⓔ

Serves 4   See photograph, page 111

4 bananas   *60–85 g/2–3 oz brown sugar*
45 g/1½ oz Tomor margarine

Preheat oven to 180 °C/350 °F/gas 4.

Peel bananas and lay them in a fireproof dish. Sprinkle with 2 tbsp water. Cover each banana with several dots of Tomor margarine and sugar. Bake for 30 minutes.

Serve with goat's or ewe's milk yoghurt or nut cream (see page 110).

Gingered-up pears

Serves 2   See photograph, page 83

2 pears
15 g/½ oz fresh root ginger, peeled and
finely chopped

1 tbsp demerara sugar
blanched almonds

Halve the pears lengthways and carefully remove the core. Arrange in the bottom of a medium size pan, cut surface uppermost, pour over 60 ml/2 fl oz water and add a quarter of the ginger. Gently simmer with the lid on until the pears are just softening. Lift them out carefully, place in serving dishes and keep warm.

To the juice in the pan add the rest of the ginger, 150 ml/¼ pint water and the sugar. Simmer for 5 minutes, then sieve.

Decorate the pears with the almonds, and serve the hot ginger sauce separately.

Fruit crumble

Serves 4

60 g/2 oz ground rice
60 g/2 oz rice flour
or
120 g/4 oz sago flour
or
60 g/2 oz rice flour
60 g/2 oz soya flour

with
60 g/2 oz Tomor margarine
60 g/2 oz brown sugar
450 g/1 lb any fruit, eg, apples,
pears, plums

Rub Tomor into flour intil it resembles fine breadcrumbs. Mix in the sugar.

Wash and slice up the fruit, put in an ovenproof dish and add a little sugar if necessary.

Place the crumbs on top of the fruit and bake in oven at 190 °C/375 °F/gas 5 until brown on top.

Millet crisp

Serves 4

60 g/2 oz Tomor margarine
60 g/2 oz soft brown sugar
120 g/4 oz millet flakes
450 g/1 lb apples and sultanas with
cinnamon
or

plums and sugar
or
rhubarb and dates
or
bananas and figs

Cream the Tomor and sugar together. Mix in the millet flakes. Place on top of chosen fruit and bake in oven at 190 °C/375 °F/gas 5 until brown on top.

Nut cream

Serves 2

60 g/2 oz mixed nuts

Grind nuts finely using the fine attachment on the mincer, or a coffee grinder. Mix with enough cold water to form a cream.
Use as cream on fruit, salads or vegetables.

NB By using different types of nuts the flavour of the cream can be varied.

Treacle toffee

Makes 250 g/9 oz

150 g/5 oz demerara sugar   *1½ tsp black treacle*
30 g/1 oz Tomor margarine   *1½ tsp golden syrup*
⅛ tsp cream of tartar

Dissolve the sugar in 50 ml/2 fl oz water, using a heavy large pan over a low heat. Add the other ingredients and bring to the boil. Do not stir the mixture. Boil to 132 °C/250 °F (when a blob dropped into cold water separates into threads that are hard but not brittle). Pour into greased tin. Cut into squares as it cools.

Peppermint creams

Makes 60

450 g/1 lb granulated sugar   *peppermint essence to taste*
⅛ tsp cream of tartar

Put 150 ml/¼ pint water and the sugar in heavy-based aluminium pan and heat gently until the sugar has dissolved. Bring to the boil, add the cream of tartar and continue boiling the mixture to 116 °C/235 °F. To check the temperature, either use a thermometer, or wait until a blob of mixture dropped into very cold water forms a soft ball, which flattens on being removed from the water.
 Pour the mixture into a cool, large flat ovenproof flan dish or on to a marble slab. Work it back and forwards in a figure of eight with a wooden spoon or spatula, adding peppermint essence as desired. The mixture will gradually become opaque and firm. Making sure your hands are very clean, not to discolour the mixture, knead until of suitable consistency to roll into individual sweets. Form into a sausage shape about 2.5 cm/1 in in diameter and slice into discs about ½ cm/¼ in thick.

Baked bananas with nut cream (*top*, see page 108 and above), Peppermint creams (*centre*), Peach condé (*bottom*, see page 107)

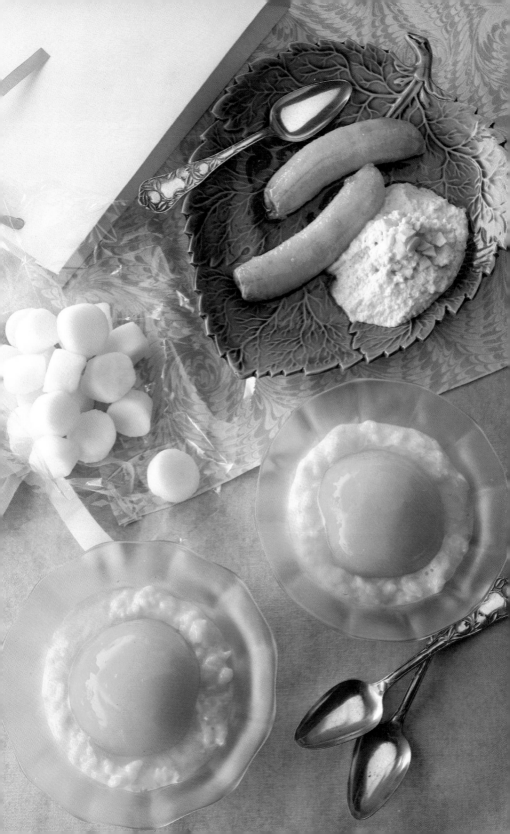

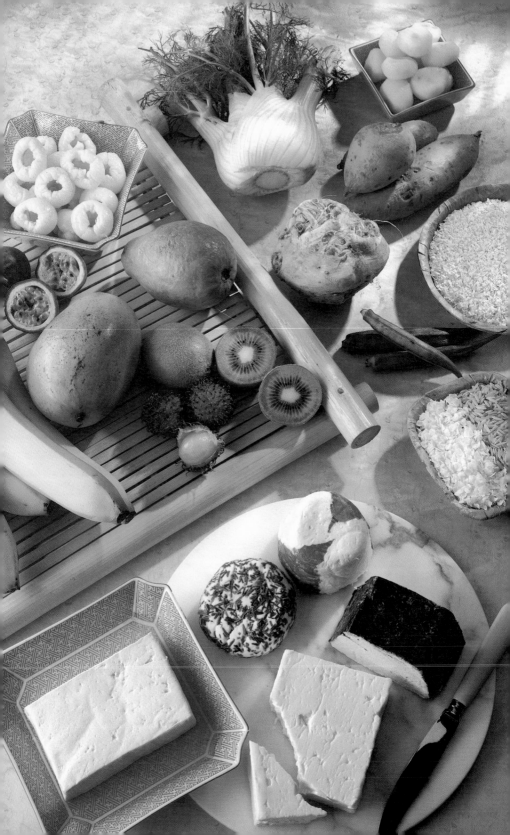

APPENDIX: FOOD LABELLING

The following serial numbers may be used on food labels in the UK as alternatives to the names of additives.

Serial number	Name of additive
E 100	curcumin
E 101	riboflavin or lactoflavin
E 102	tartrazine
E 104	quinoline yellow
E 110	sunset yellow FCF or orange yellow S
E 120	cochineal or carminic acid
E 122	carmoisine or azorubine
E 123	amaranth
E 124	ponceau 4R or cochineal red A
E 127	erythrosine BS
E 131	patent blue V
E 132	indigo carmine or indigotine
E 140	chlorophyll
E 141	copper complexes of chlorophyll and chlorophyllins
E 142	green S or acid brilliant green BS or lissamine green
E 150	caramel
E 151	black PN or brilliant black BN
E 153	carbon black or vegetable carbon
E 160(a)	alpha-carotene, beta-carotene, gamma-carotene
E 160(b)	annatto, bixin, norbixin
E 160(c)	capsanthin or capsorubin
E 160(d)	lycopene
E 160(e)	beta-apo-8'-carotenal (C30)
E 160(f)	ethyl ester of beta-apo-8'-carotenoic acid (C30)
E 161(a)	flavoxanthin
E 161(b)	lutein
E 161(c)	cryptoxanthin
E 161(d)	rubixanthin
E 161(e)	violaxanthin
E 161(f)	rhodoxanthin
E 161(g)	canthaxanthin
E 162	beetroot red or betanin
E 163	anthocyanins
E 170	calcium carbonate
E 171	titanium dioxide
E 172	iron oxide and hydroxides
E 173	aluminium
E 174	silver
E 175	gold
E 180	pigment rubine or lithol rubine BK
E 200	sorbic acid
E 201	sodium sorbate

Allergy-free foods: (*clockwise*) Bananas, mango, guava, passion fruit, lychees, kiwi fruit, fennel, water chestnuts, sweet potato, celeriac, millet, okra, flaked and brown rice, selection of goat's cheese, feta, soya cheese

E 202	potassium sorbate
E 203	calcium sorbate
E 210	benzoic acid
E 211	sodium benzoate
E 212	potassium benzoate
E 213	calcium benzoate
E 214	ethyl 4-hydroxybenzoate
E 215	ethyl 4-hydroxybenzoate sodium salt
E 216	propyl 4-hydroxybenzoate
E 217	propyl 4-hydroxybenzoate sodium salt
E 218	methyl 4-hydroxybenzoate
E 219	methyl 4-hydroxybenzoate sodium salt
E 220	sulphur dioxide
E 221	sodium sulphite
E 222	sodium hydrogen sulphite
E 223	sodium metabisulphite
E 224	potassium metabisulphite
E 226	calcium sulphite
E 227	calcium hydrogen sulphite
E 230	biphenyl or diphenyl
E 231	2-hydroxybiphenyl
E 232	sodium biphenyl-2-yl-oxide
E 233	2-(thiazol-4-yl) benzimidazole
E 236	formic acid
E 237	sodium formate
E 238	calcium formate
E 239	hexamine
E 249	potassium nitrite
E 250	sodium nitrite
E 251	sodium nitrate
E 252	potassium nitrate
E 260	acetic acid
E 261	potassium acetate
E 262	sodium hydrogen diacetate
E 263	calcium acetate
E 270	lactic acid
E 280	propionic acid
E 281	sodium propionate
E 282	calcium propionate
E 283	potassium propionate
E 290	carbon dioxide
E 300	L-ascorbic acid
E 301	sodium-L-ascorbate
E 302	calcium-L-ascorbate
E 304	6-0-palmitoyl-L-ascorbic acid
E 306	extracts of natural origin rich in tocopherols
E 307	synthetic alpha-tocopherol
E 308	synthetic gamma-tocopherol
E 309	synthetic delta-tocopherol
E 310	propyl gallate
E 311	octyl gallate
E 312	dodecyl gallate
E 320	butylated hydroxyanisole
E 321	butylated hydroxytoluene

E 322	lecithins
E 325	sodium lactate
E 326	potassium lactate
E 327	calcium lactate
E 330	citric acid
E 331	sodium dihydrogen citrate
E 331	disodium citrate
E 331	trisodium citrate
E 332	potassium dihydrogen citrate
E 332	tripotassium citrate
E 333	calcium citrate
E 333	dicalcium citrate
E 333	tricalcium citrate
E 334	tartaric acid
E 335	sodium tartrate
E 336	potassium tartrate
E 336	potassium hydrogen tartrate
E 337	potassium sodium tartrate
E 338	orthophosphoric acid
E 339(a)	sodium dihydrogen orthophosphate
E 339(b)	disodium hydrogen orthophosphate
E 339(c)	trisodium orthophosphate
E 340(a)	potassium dihydrogen orthophosphate
E 340(b)	dipotassium hydrogen orthophosphate
E 340(c)	tripotassium orthophosphate
E 341(a)	calcium tetrahydrogen diorthophosphate
E 341(b)	calcium hydrogen orthophosphate
E 341(c)	tricalcium diorthophosphate
E 400	alginic acid
E 401	sodium alginate
E 402	potassium alginate
E 403	ammonium alginate
E 404	calcium alginate
E 405	propane-1,2-diol alginate
E 406	agar
E 407	carrageenan
E 410	locust bean gum
E 412	guar gum
E 413	tragacanth
E 414	acacia or gum arabic
E 415	xanthan gum
E 420(i)	sorbitol
E 420(ii)	sorbitol syrup
E 421	mannitol
E 422	glycerol
E 440(a)	pectin
E 440(b)	pectin, amidated
E 450(a)	disodium dihydrogen diphosphate
E 450(a)	tetrasodium diphosphate
E 450(a)	tetrapotassium diphosphate
E 450(a)	trisodium diphosphate
E 450(b)	pentasodium triphosphate
E 450(b)	pentapotassium triphosphate
E 450(c)	sodium polyphosphate

E 450(c)	potassium polyphosphates
E 460(i)	microcrystalline cellulose
E 460(ii)	powdered cellulose
E 461	methylcellulose
E 463	hydroxypropylcellulose
E 464	hydroxypropylmethylcellulose
E 465	ethylmethylcellulose
E 466	carboxymethylcellulose, sodium salt
E 470	sodium potassium and calcium salts of fatty acids
E 471	mono- and di-glycerides of fatty acids
E 472(a)	acetic acid esters of mono- and di-glycerides of fatty acids
E 472(b)	lactic acid esters of mono- and di-glycerides of fatty acids
E 472(c)	citric acid esters of mono- and di-glycerides of fatty acids
E 472(d)	tartaric acid esters of mono- and di-glycerides of fatty acids
E 472(e)	diacetyltartaric acid esters of mono- and di-glycerides of fatty acids
E 473	sucrose esters of fatty acids
E 474	sucroglycerides
E 475	polyglycerol esters of fatty acids
E 477	propane-1, 2-diol esters of fatty acids
E 481	sodium stearoyl-2-lactylate
E 482	calcium stearoyl-2-lactylate
E 483	stearyl tartrate

People with further interest should consult the leaflet called *Look at the Label* published by the Ministry of Agriculture, Fisheries and Food, and the British Food Manufacturing Industries Research Association publication, *Food Additives*.

Since they have hardly ever produced symptoms, substances denoted by the following E numbers are permitted on the first stage of the exclusion diet.

E 100	E 300	E 421
E 101	E 301	E 422
E 120	E 302	E 440(a)
E 140	E 306	E 440(b)
E 150	E 307	E 460(i)
E 153	E 308	E 460(ii)
E 160a	E 309	E 466
E 160b	E 322	E 500
E 160c	E 336	E 501
E 160d	E 363	E 504
E 161a	E 375	E 508
E 161b	E 400	E 509
E 161c	E 404	E 515
E 161d	E 406	E 516
E 161e	E 407	E 518

E 161f	E 410	E 529
E 161g	E 412	E 530
E 162	E 413	E 542
E 170	E 414	E 559
E 172	E 415	E 901
E 290	E 416	E 903
E 296	E 420(i)	E 904
E 297	E 420(ii)	

ACKNOWLEDGEMENTS

The authors would like to thank their families for putting up with them and for tasting the recipes, and Alison Wilson for keeping them sane and organized during the writing of this book.

1984   Elizabeth Workman, Virginia Alun Jones and
                                                        John Hunter

The publishers are grateful to the following for their help in the preparation of this book: the photographs were taken by Peter Myers, assisted by Neil Mersh; art direction was by Rose and Lamb Design Partnership, styling by Penny Markham and food preparation by Lisa Collard.

INDEX

Page numbers in *italic* refer to the illustrations.

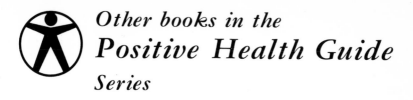

Other books in the
Positive Health Guide
Series

THE HIGH-FIBRE
COOKBOOK
Recipes for Good Health
Pamela Westland
Introduction by Dr Denis
Burkitt

DON'T FORGET FIBRE IN
YOUR DIET
*To help avoid many of our commonest
diseases*
Dr Denis Burkitt

ENJOY SEX IN THE MIDDLE
YEARS
*Published in association with the National
Marriage Guidance Council*
Dr Christine Sandford

GET A BETTER NIGHT'S
SLEEP
Prof Ian Oswald and Dr Kirstine
Adam

THE BACK – RELIEF FROM
PAIN
*Patterns of back pain – how to deal with
and avoid them*
Dr Alan Stoddard

BEAT HEART DISEASE!
*A cardiologist explains how you can help
your heart and enjoy a healthier life*
Prof Ristéard Mulcahy

HIGH BLOOD PRESSURE
*What it means for you, and how to
control it*
Dr Eoin O'Brien and Prof Kevin
O'Malley

THE DIABETICS'
DIET BOOK
A new high-fibre eating programme
Dr Jim Mann and the Oxford
Dietetic Group

STRESS AND RELAXATION
*Self-help ways to cope with stress and
relieve nervous tension, ulcers, insomnia,
migraine and high blood pressure*
Jane Madders

VARICOSE VEINS
*How they are treated, and what you can do
to help*
Prof Harold Ellis

ECZEMA AND DERMATITIS
How to cope with inflamed skin
Prof Rona MacKie

ANXIETY AND DEPRESSION
A practical guide to recovery
Prof Robert Priest

ACNE
Advice on clearing your skin
Prof Ronald Marks

OVERCOMING DYSLEXIA
A straightforward guide for families and teachers
Dr Bevé Hornsby

EYES
Their problems and treatments
Michael Glasspool, FRCS

CONQUERING PAIN
How to overcome the discomfort of arthritis, backache, migraine, heart disease, childbirth, period pains and many other common conditions
Dr Sampson Lipton

ASTHMA AND HAY FEVER
How to relieve wheezing and sneezing
Dr Allan Knight

OVERCOMING ARTHRITIS
A guide to coping with stiff or aching joints
Dr Frank Dudley Hart

PSORIASIS
A guide to one of the commonest skin diseases
Prof Ronald Marks

DIABETES
A practical new guide to healthy living
Dr Jim Anderson